The Book on Puberty for Girls
The Complete Guide for young Girls and their Parents

By Flora J. Blair & Brian Mahoney

Table of Contents

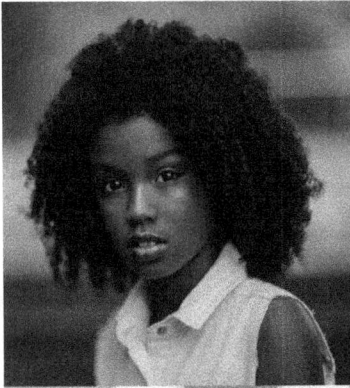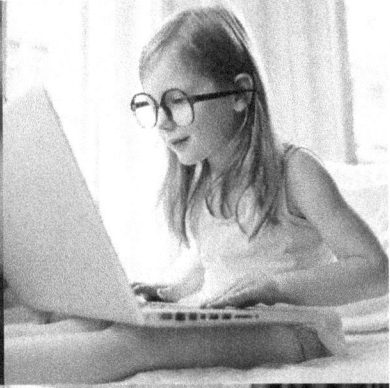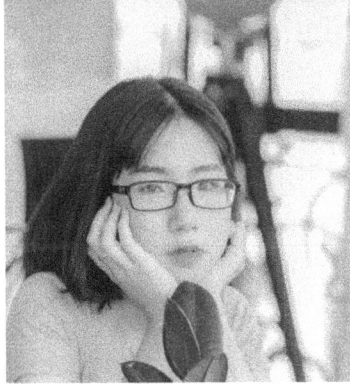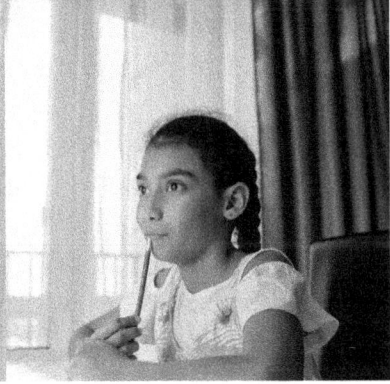

Introduction

Thank you for picking up this book. Just by reading it, you are a change-maker! By putting it into practice, you might change your life, and the life of the girls you reach.

Knowledge is power, and knowing all about your body's changes will make you an expert on your body. I know you picked up this book to learn about Puberty for yourself. But if you read something you don't understand or want to know more about, I strongly encourage you to share those questions with a trusted adult. You are a beautiful, powerful, smart girl who feels confident about her body and her life. Puberty doesn't change that. If anything, Puberty is an opportunity to feel even more confident and assertive in your body. Why? Because you are becoming a guru on its awesomeness!

You may have learned some information in your health class at school but still have many more questions. As your body changes, you will have new questions about what is happening. I hope you will use this book as a reliable reference to help answer your questions.

Throughout this book, we will discuss some key questions you might have about Puberty and body changes. We'll start by discussing what Puberty is (the regular body changes that signal your transition into adulthood). Next, we'll talk about some of the body changes you might expect during this time, starting with the small changes (Hey, how did that hair get there?), and then we will discuss the bigger ones like breast development and menstruation.

Introduction

We'll even talk about how you can navigate issues like health, well-being, emotions, and privacy. In each section, we'll highlight what physical changes you may notice, as well as share tips about how to care for your body as these changes happen. Puberty is a thrilling time filled with new opportunities to understand your body even better.

When we equip ourselves with correct information, we have everything we need to move into adulthood, confident that our incredible bodies have all they need to help us live an extraordinary life!

The first thing to know about growing up, is that you don't need to have it all figured out. It's okay to learn as you go. Even when you get older and gain more responsibility, never worry about having everything perfectly under control.

Face it: No captain of a ship, knows every little detail of their journey ahead of time. The truth is that life is a beautiful challenge, changes and all. If any of it gets overwhelming, stay confident that it will only be temporary. Think about all the great things you have going on right now. Puberty won't change that. It will change you, but it won't change the fact that you can remain healthy and happy through adolescence. I know this because I am a Health Education teacher. I work with hundreds of students each year to manage the time of life between childhood and adulthood.

Introduction

For girls working their way through middle school, I help them successfully handle accurate information, valuable resources, and a whole bunch of humor.

Plus, I think I have a knack for simply listening and understanding what kids are going through. We have a lot of fun in my classes because health and wellness are all about students themselves. I'm guessing that is why you picked up this book—it's all about you! Smart move, my friend.

I hope that this book enables mothers, fathers, aunts, grandparents, godparents, sisters, and women in your life to support your girls and to make a difference for them. When those girls are older and perhaps have children of their own, I hope that they will do the same, sharing from the role models they had.

So let's learn together about this adventure called Puberty. It may not be fun all the time, but being prepared means, you can be ready for the changes that lie ahead.

Let's get you prepared for the journey of your remarkable body. Because here is the thing: We get only one body—so let's love it, understand it, and take care of it.

DEDICATION

This book is dedicated to my Sisters
Beth-Ann, Rachel, Leslie & Susan
Blessings from God

ACKNOWLEDGMENTS

I WOULD LIKE TO ACKNOWLEDGE ALL THE HARD WORK OF THE MEN AND WOMEN OF THE UNITED STATES MILITARY, WHO RISK THEIR LIVES ON A DAILY BASIS, TO MAKE THE WORLD A SAFER PLACE.

Disclaimer

This book was written as a guide and for information purposes only. This book is not meant to take the place of legal or medical professional advice. If advice is needed in any of these fields, you are advised to seek the services of a professional.

While the author has attempted to make the information in this book as accurate as possible, no guarantee is given as to the accuracy or currency of any individual item. Laws and procedures related to business, health and well being are constantly changing.

Therefore, in no event shall Brian Mahoney, the author of this book be liable for any special, indirect, or consequential damages or any damages whatsoever in connection with the use of the information herein provided.

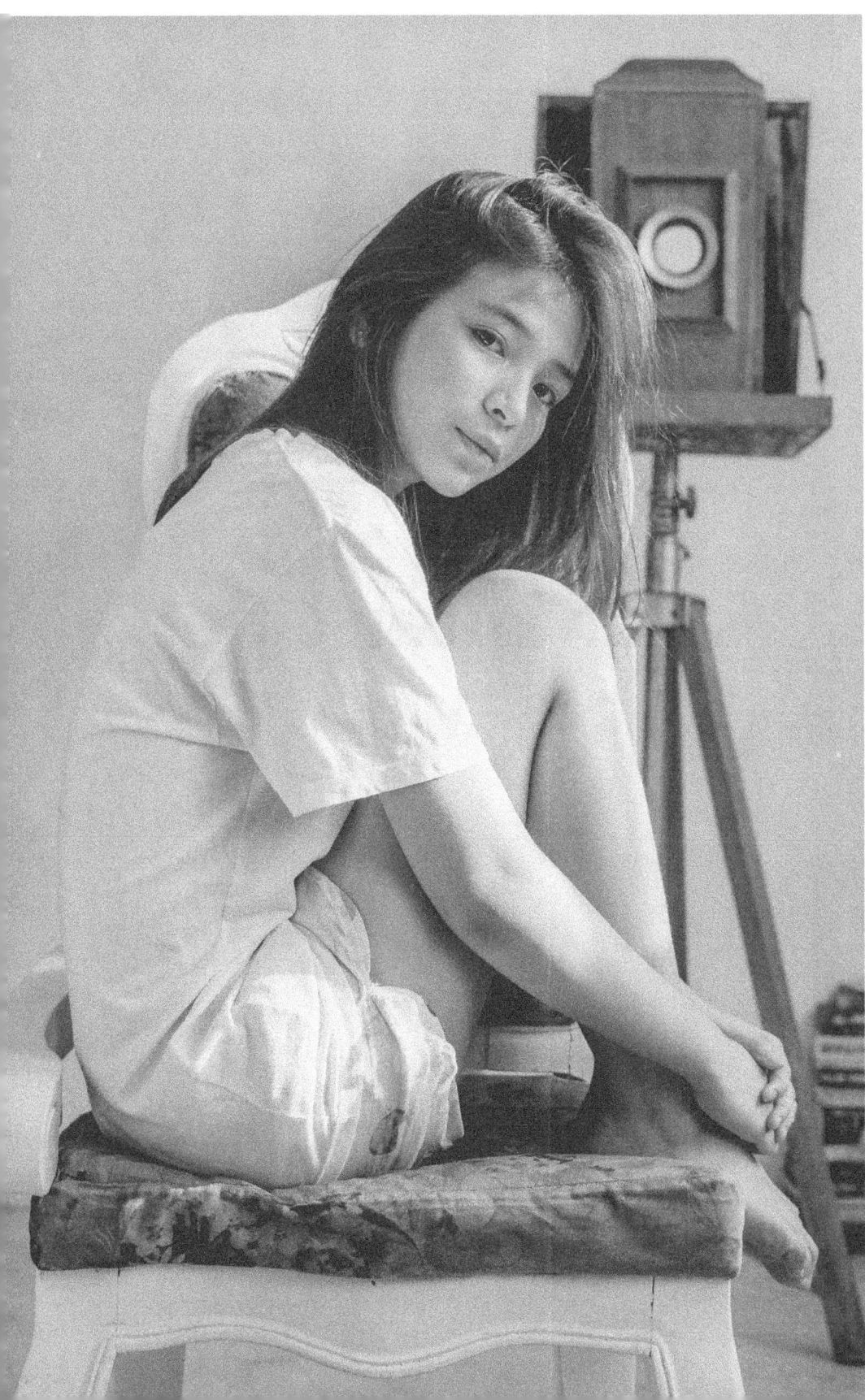

Chapter One:
Puberty for Girls

Puberty for Girls

Puberty is a necessary period in every person's life; It is the time in life when a person develops from a child into an adult. It is a period of physical growth when the body sexually matures and becomes able to reproduce.

It is significantly vital to get the correct information at this particular time. It will help you form your habits and develop skills to maintain your health. The puberty period is significant for your future life.

Puberty is the time when you experience physical, hormonal, and emotional changes and rapidly approach adulthood. These changes prepare your organism for conception and giving birth. Of course, it doesn't mean that you are ready to be a mother. Puberty manifests that it is high time to say goodbye to childhood. The realization that soon your body will face significant changes can cause both joy and sadness.

Just as people have different personalities, their bodies can be programmed to go through Puberty at different times, too. Your older sister may start Puberty after you, or your best friend may start changing years before you. And this is all NORMAL. The most important thing to remember is that Puberty begins when your body decides it's the right time for you.

Puberty for Girls

There will be many changes during Puberty that you can see happening when you look in the mirror. Your body will grow in all directions—up, down, and all around. You will grow taller and get a curvier shape. Another significant change will be to your privates. You will develop hair in places where you didn't have it before (like your vulva, armpits, and legs). Your breasts will start to grow bigger. Your skin will even begin to change; it can get sweatier and oilier.

Puberty also causes changes to your body that you can't see in the mirror. Just as your body is growing and changing shape, so is your brain. You are becoming older and wiser, and the way you think will start to change. You may notice that you feel much more emotional than you did in the past. We like to say that in Puberty, you can feel like the whole emoji keyboard in just a few short minutes.

Is there a point to all of this? Yes! Going through Puberty means your body will become capable of reproducing. It's preparing to be able to grow another human. The way your body prepares for this is through a necessary process called menstruation, or getting your period. Everybody has to go through Puberty because we would become extinct like the dinosaurs if we didn't.

Puberty happens gradually over many years. You will not just wake up one day and magically transform from a kid into an adult. It makes the changes more straightforward to get used to.

Puberty for Girls

First Signs of Puberty

You may be asking yourself, "How in the world will I know that I have started puberty?" The answer is this: All you have to do is listen to your body—it will start dropping some hints that your journey has begun.

Your ovaries, which are parts of your body that produce hormones, will begin signaling that it's time for all the other changes to start. It is during this time that you may grow taller or curvier than you were before. This sudden burst of bigger is called a growth spurt, and let us talk more about it.

Growth Spurt

One other early sign that Puberty is about to start in girls is growth spurts. Girls may get anywhere between two and eight inches or more in the puberty period. They generally cease from growing two years following the start of their menstruation. The female's hands and feet grow wider as well as longer. The feet might grow more rapidly or stop growing before noticing additional puberty changes.

When a girl gets taller during Puberty, this is the first noticeable sign that she experiences this period. It, however, is merely the beginning. Generally, by age fourteen, the spine growing process has ended. Besides, the pelvis bones widen and smooth out to accommodate childbirth. It may happen up to eighteen years of age or later.

Puberty for Girls

Up Next ... Breasts

Remember those hormones that started signaling the rest of your body to board the puberty train? Well, they have also sent a message to your breasts to begin growing. The first thing you may notice is some soreness or tenderness and a hard bump just underneath your nipple. The bump may make the dark circles around your nipples (called your areola) look more oversized or puffy. The hard lump is called a breast bud, and it is the first sign of budding breasts.

For most girls, when the breasts start to grow, this period is most exciting. However, this phase frequently causes anxiety and many worries, such as the large size they will become, whether they will look good or not, and whether or not they will be healthy. To quell some of the worries, here is some basic information relating to healthy breasts.

Breast 'buds' that are generally tender is usually the initial sign that Puberty has started in girls. Some girls will notice their breasts' growth from as young as seven to eight years of age. Others will not begin until about age thirteen. The breast growth timing is decided by the individual personal biological 'clock,' which tells the body to start producing high amounts of feminine hormones. The breasts proceed through five phases of growth for five or six years and continue until full maturity is attained at age seventeen to eighteen.

Puberty for Girls

The makeup of the blood includes milk ducts and glands, fat and connective tissue. For young women and teenagers, the breast tissue is dense and firm and then gets fattier and softer as the female ages. The breasts do not have muscle tissue in them, which is why no exercise is designed to enlarge them. However, muscles found beneath the breasts, the pectoral muscles, may be firmed or compressed to offer shape and lift. It is similar to the 'pecs' generally found on the bodies of bodybuilders.

The breasts of a woman, as designed by nature, produce milk so that babies can feed. However, in society, the breasts are usually seen as a feminine symbol and sexually attractive. Therefore, it is not surprising that young women will have a lot of questions about the breast.

Body Hair

Just as your body is starting to grow breasts, other weird changes are happening. You might notice hair growing in places where you hadn't seen any before. You might have always had baby-soft hair on your legs, the kind of hair that is almost invisible – but suddenly, that hair is becoming darker and thicker. You will also notice hair under your arms. Even your eyebrows may begin to look thicker.

You will start to see hair in your private areas, too. It is called pubic hair, and it is something everyone gets. It is caused by all those hormones kicking in and trying to take your body into adulthood.

Puberty for Girls

Some people get very little hair growth, while others have a lot. Like many things, everybody is different. Some girls accept their hair, while others don't like it. If you are fine with your new hair, this is a personal choice, don't worry about it.

Hair Removal Tips

Suppose you don't like the new hair on your body. In that case, millions of people remove hair from their bodies every day. Now you will join the ranks of those familiar with razors, shaving cream, depilatory creams, and other methods of keeping the hair under control. But how do you know which method is suitable for you?

The most common method of hair removal is the old-fashioned razor and shaving cream. Many girls like it because it is quick and easy. If you're going to go this route, be sure to get a good shaving cream that has a moisturizer in it to help keep your skin soft. Only use a sharp razor, as a dull one can lead to nicks and cuts. Go slowly at first until you know how the razor feels in your hand. It's not something to rush!

A depilatory cream is another option. These creams are available in the shaving aisle at your local store. They work by dissolving the hair so that when you wash away the cream, the hair goes with it. These creams work very well for some girls, but for others, they are a disappointment. Beware if you have susceptible skin!

Puberty for Girls

Try using it on just a tiny spot first to make sure you don't have any breakouts from the chemicals in the cream.

There are other options for removing body hair. Some women get their unwanted hair waxed off. You can do this at home, but it can be excruciating. Some options are permanent and very expensive, like electrolysis. If you're curious about any of these possibilities, talk to your parents about them. Remember, if your new hair doesn't worry you, then it shouldn't bother anybody else. You don't have to remove it.

Period Please

Usually, once you have begun to develop breasts and pubic hair, it is a sign that you may soon get your period. Some girls get their period at younger ages, like 9 or 10 years old. Other girls may start when they are older, sometimes as old as 15 or 16. There may be lots of chatter at school among the girls about who got their period first. But ovaries can't race, and getting your period is not a competition. Whenever your period starts, it will be the right time for you.

Puberty for Girls

Change of shape

Girls and boys generally have a physique that is quite similar before Puberty. However, both sexes have transformed shape that is noticeable and distinct from each other as sex hormones increase. For the girls, the transformation stage is not so pronounced. Instead, estrogen, the sex hormone of the female, encourages fat to lie down. This fat is focused on the bust as well as hips and is quite normal. It will not be so noticeable in girls that frequently exercise.

The new face

When the teenage girl experiences increased height and body fat, the face bones also experience growth. The changes are not so dramatic as with the boys; however, appearances change while the face gets more angular and longer.

Pimples and Acne

One of the concerns girls often have during Puberty is whether they will get acne (also known as pimples). What you should know is that Puberty does not have to doom you to a life of acne cream and zits. While you may get some acne during this time, having a good skincare routine can help keep breakouts to a minimum. But pimples are indeed another part of Puberty that many of us have to go through.

Puberty for Girls

When your body begins producing the hormones that signal Puberty to start, you also start making extra oil inside your body. That excess oil often mixes with sweat and dirt and can clog your pores (tiny openings on your skin). Those clogged pores cause acne and blackheads.

Washing your face daily with a gentle cleanser and following up with a moisturizer should help clear away much of the bacteria that causes acne. If you find that you are having a more severe breakout, you may want to go to the drugstore with a trusted adult and purchase some anti-acne cream with a bit of medicine in it. Be sure to look for oil and soap-free since it is better for your skin.

Always wash after exercising. Physical activity can send those oil glands into an even higher overdrive! It's always good to shower after the workout, and if you make a facial cleanser part of your routine, it should become an easy thing to remember.
If you are a girl, when you choose makeup, make sure it's the kind that doesn't clog pores. These are often called hypoallergenic. When you are at home, wash off the makeup and go natural.

Whatever you do, don't squeeze the pimples to make them go away. It might be tempting to do this, but you could make the problem worse. Squeezing a pimple can force the infection further into the skin, leading to even more acne or scarring.

Puberty for Girls

Sometimes skin breakouts can become more severe than drugstore treatments can manage. If you are experiencing difficult acne that won't go away, ask an adult to take you to see a dermatologist (skin doctor). He or she can give you more potent medicine to help with breakouts.

Let's dispel some myths about acne. First, it is not caused by dirty skin. Acne can happen to someone who has a flawless face and body. Things like chocolate, candies, or soda don't drive it. It isn't caused by anything like that at all.

There is no way to predict who will get acne and who won't. If some of your relatives had acne, the odds of you getting it are a bit higher. But even those who have no history of acne in the family could wind up with a bad case of it. You can't even be sure where it's going to happen – some get acne on their face, but others wind up with it on their shoulders, backs, or chest. It's thanks to all those hormones going wild – you just never know what is going to happen!

Body Odor

One day you may come home after running around playing and find yourself saying, "What is that smell?" only to realize it's you. You have just discovered you are developing body odor. Remember that your body produces increased hormones, and there are new sweat glands under your arms, feet, and between your legs. This combination can sometimes be a little smelly.

Puberty for Girls

But body odor is a common part of Puberty, and with good hygiene practices, you can come out smelling like a rose!

You sweat and create bacteria every single day, so you will need to wash your body daily. Pay special attention to your underarms, feet, and genitals. You can buy different types of deodorants or antiperspirants to counter body odor under your arms. Deodorants will not keep you from sweating, but they will keep the sweat from being stinky. Be sure not to use too much, as many people can be sensitive to deodorant chemicals. Antiperspirants keep your body from producing sweat. You should only use antiperspirants under your arms. Sweat is a necessary function of your body, and without it, you can become overheated or even get sick.

What Is Normal?

One of the most common questions girls ask about all the changes happening during Puberty is, "Hey, is this normal?" Here is the short answer to that question: Yes! Your body will experience all sorts of new sensations and functions during this vital time in your life. Growing very quickly or watching your body change shape may feel unusual. You may not even enjoy some of the changes that come with Puberty. It is all okay.

Puberty for Girls

Puberty for Girls

While your body changes are similar to the changes happening in other girls' bodies your age, your body is unique because it is all yours. It means that your puberty experience will be sort of normal. Being different is normal!

The more you trust and listen to your body, the easier it will tell if something needs special attention. For example, if something in your body feels painful or uncomfortable during this time, you should talk to a trusted adult about it right away.

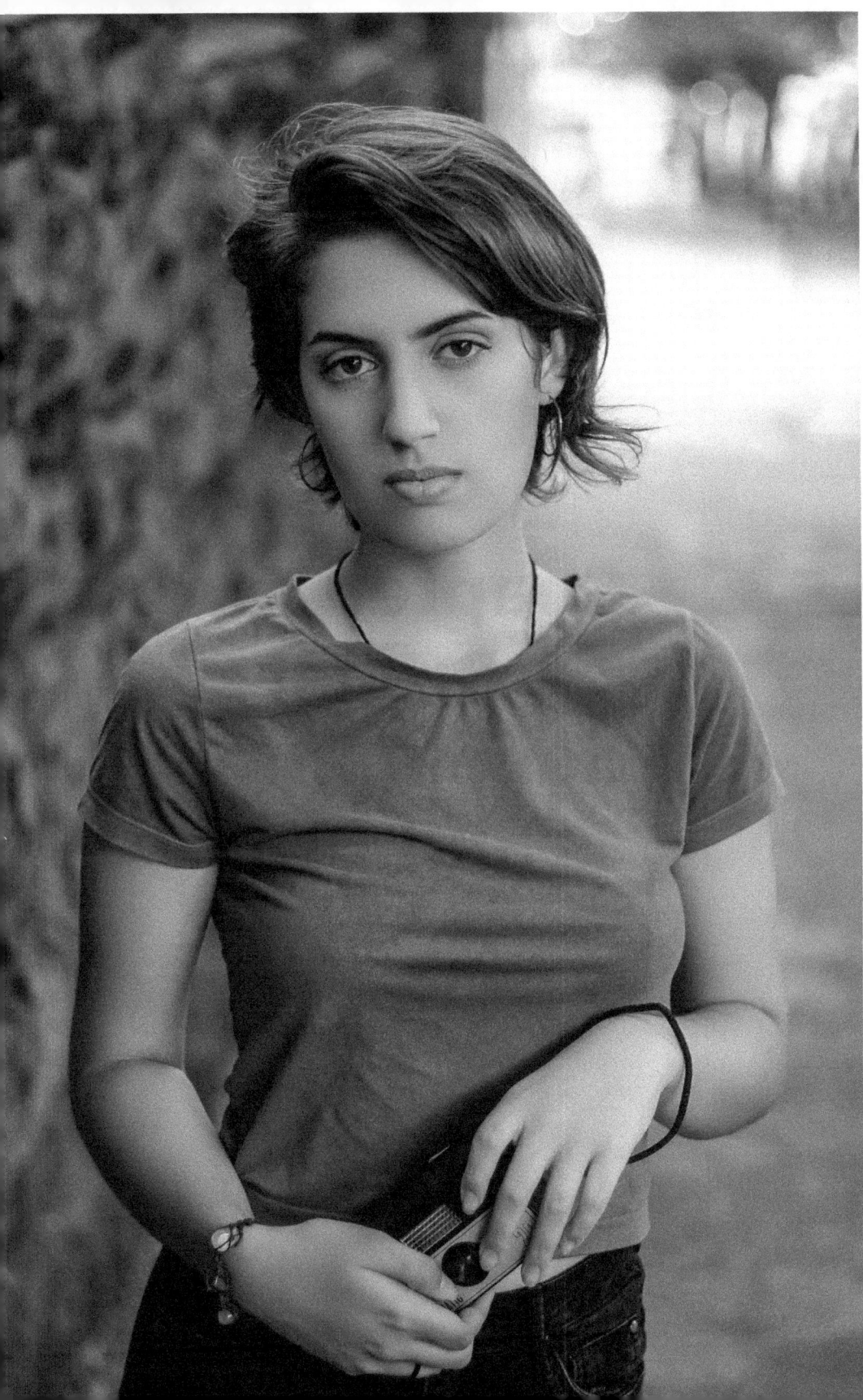

Chapter Two: Breast development and Bras

Breast Development and Bras

Breast development is one of the body changes that put puberty front and center, but it doesn't happen overnight. There are five stages of breast development, and they occur over several years. Whether you are about to dive into stage 1 or are swimming in stage 3, here is what you should know about your breasts as they grow and change.

When do breasts start growing?

Many breasts will begin to develop as early as age 8 or as late as age 13. Breasts of some girls grow gradually, while others grow rapidly. Some girls may feel like their breasts never begin to grow. But, at various ages and different levels, girls start to flourish. At 12, one girl may have more developed breasts while her friend might still be flat as a board.

The size of breasts attracts a lot of attention, and many girls question how they can boost their breasts. There is no magical cream or a pill that would accelerate the process or make breasts bigger. Heredity identifies the breast size of a girl. If your mother has big or small breasts, then expect the same size.

These are the stages of breast development that you will encounter:

Stage 1 Preadolescent Breasts

Around 8 to 11 years old

Breast Development and Bras

Before we start talking about how breasts grow, we should begin where we all begin. You already have nipples. Nipples are the small buttons of skin on top of your areolae, those darker circles on your chest. Your nipples may be flat or pointy. Sometimes they start flat but become erect when it's cold outside—they are sensitive little things! Nipples have tiny holes in them you cannot see, and those itty-bitty holes will one day release the milk humans make to feed new babies. Yes, just like cows, humans make milk, too! All mammals make milk.

Stage 2 Breast Buds

Around 10 to 11½ years old

If you remember from chapter 1, the first thing you may notice as you begin breast development is a hard, nickel-size lump just underneath your nipple called a breast bud. Breast buds form when the breast tissue and milk glands begin to grow. Breast buds can be so tiny that you might not even notice they are there. But they can make your breast area sore and tender.

If you feel some slight discomfort, don't worry. It is just your breasts doing what they are supposed to do. You may have breast buds of completely different sizes, or you may have a bud in one breast but not in the other. How your breasts will grow cannot be compared with any of your friends. Your experience will be all your own, so don't let anyone tell you how your breasts "should" look. Breast development is different for every girl.

Breast Development and Bras

Your body knows what it is doing, even when that looks different from what other people's bodies are doing.

Stage 3 Breast Growth

Around 11½ to 13 years old

After you have developed breast buds, your breasts will begin to grow more fatty tissue and milk glands. At this stage, you may notice that your breasts are slightly cone-shaped. During this time, you may also realize that your areolae are getting bigger and puffier. These signs mean your puberty train is on the right track.

Stage 4 Onset of Puberty

Around 13 to 15 years old

During this stage, your breasts will begin to lose the cone shape they developed in stage 3 and start to take on the size and shape of the breasts you will have in adulthood. The changes to your breast shape in this stage are mainly caused by a hormone called estrogen. Estrogen is the body's puberty boss, telling it when it is time to go to work and when the job is done—estrogen bosses around lots of other parts of Puberty besides your breasts.

Breast Development and Bras

Stage 5 Mature Breasts

Around 15 and older

Stage 5 is the final stage of puberty breast development. Your breasts have reached maturity at this stage and are the size and shape they will likely be in adulthood. The average girl will take three to five years to go from the first stage to the fifth stage of breast development, but it can take up to 10 years for some girls. Remember, this is a major stop on a long ride!

Getting a brassiere

A bra is an excellent solution for every girl. It is an essential thing, especially when the girl is involved in sport and exercises. Bras may protect the breast tissue and provide support for the breasts. Some ladies may even prefer the bras to smooth out their silhouettes, making them feel more relaxed. A bra will make a girl feel less vulnerable when wearing a light top, like a T-shirt.

Some girls are looking forward to wearing their first bras, but others are dreading it. Wearing a bra like something new can be challenging to adapt to. It may bag or gap while a bra is on, ride up, dig in, or pop up. The straps can slip off or dig within a girl's shoulders. And a bra can peek out the clothes of a girl.

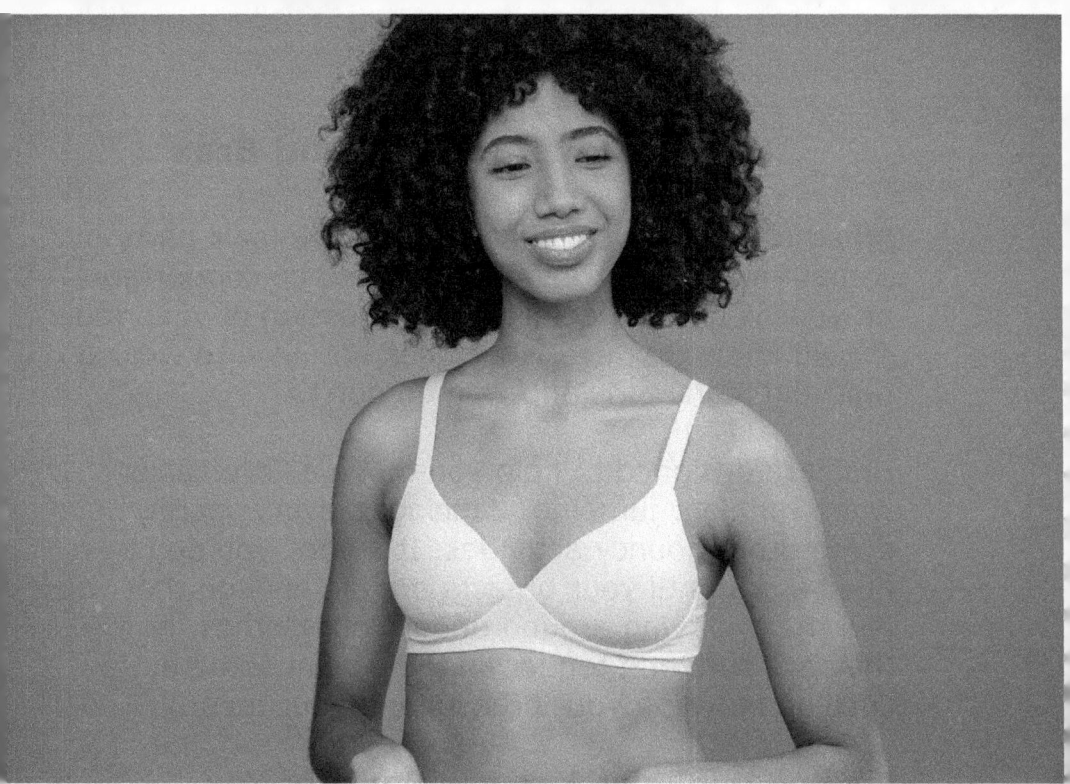

Breast Development and Bras

Whether getting your first bra is cause for a party or something you're dreading, it should be comfortable on your body and feel like an expression of you. You should know that every girl does not have to wear a bra, and many girls and women don't.

Bras are designed to help you move a little easier when running, jumping, dancing, playing sports, or doing other bouncy activities. It means you don't need a bra until your breasts are big enough that you feel them moving around under your clothes, or if they are sore and tender and you want some extra cushion between your breasts and your tops.

Finding the Right Size and Style for You

First, there are different types of bras. The first bra a girl usually has is a training bra, which doesn't provide a lot of support, but does help you get accustomed to wearing a bra. Some girls find bra-wearing itchy first, so it's best if a training bra doesn't have much lace or frills to annoy you.

As your breasts get bigger, you might be interested in other types of bras, including some that have wires (covered, of course). It helps give some structure to the bra and offers more support. A sports bra is another kind of bra that provides even more support. Sports bras usually fit snugly, so you can run around and play sports without discomfort. You don't have to be into sports to wear a sports bra, though; some girls like how they look and feel and wear them all the time!

Breast Development and Bras

Sports bras come in different sizes, small, medium, and large, but other bras have a chest size (in the US, this is measured in inches) and cup size. The cup size is usually measured from AA (smallest) to EE (largest). It is always good to get your bra size measured by an expert. Most bra stores have people called a "lingerie specialist" (which is a fancy way of saying "bra fitter") trained to tell you the right bra size for you. They will measure your breasts and around your waist over your T-shirt and help you pick out a bra that fits best. It's always a good idea to get your bras fitted, so you don't have to fight with a too tight or too loose bra. To test if you have a well-fitting bra, you should be able to comfortably fit two fingers under the bra band (the one that hooks around your back). A bra that is too tight or too loose won't provide any support, and it might even pinch you!

How Does This Thing Work?

Figuring out how to put on a bra can seem a little complicated. None of us were born with this particular skill set, so don't be afraid to ask your mom, big sister, or another trusted adult to help you out.

For the most part, there are two ways people put on bras. The first is to lean forward and slip your arms through the straps, letting your breasts fall into the cups. Once you stand up straight, you can reach around and fasten the hooks in the back.

Breast Development and Bras

You want to make sure that the back band of the bra sits just below your shoulder blades. (Some bras hook in the front, which makes the whole process easier.)

The second way is easier if you have a hard time reaching around to your back. With this method, you hold the bra upside down and inside out. Wrap the bra around you with the cups toward your back so you can fasten the hooks in front of you, and then turn the bra around and finish putting it on. Now you can adjust the straps to make sure they are comfortable. If the bra feels too tight or loose around your back, simply adjust the hooks.

Breasts and Bras Dos and Don'ts

There is a lot of information to share at this puberty stop. If your brain feels a little swirly right now, don't worry. You can always come back and reread this section. For now, here is a shortlist of the most important things to remember about bras and breasts.

Remember that your body is unique, and the timing of your breast development will be the right time for your body.

DO find a comfortable bra and a good fit.

DO measure, or get measured, so that you know what size bra you should get.

Breast Development and Bras

DO ignore everything TV and movies tell you about having breasts; they are almost always wrong.

DO trust yourself and your body. You are practically an expert on it!

DON'T try to figure it all out alone. It is more than okay to ask an adult.

DON'T compare your breasts, or any other part of your body, with other girls'. You have different genes, and your genes are great.

DON'T feel like you must wear a bra before you are ready.

Unless a trusted adult or medical professional...

DON'T listen to anyone who tells you that they know more about your body than you.

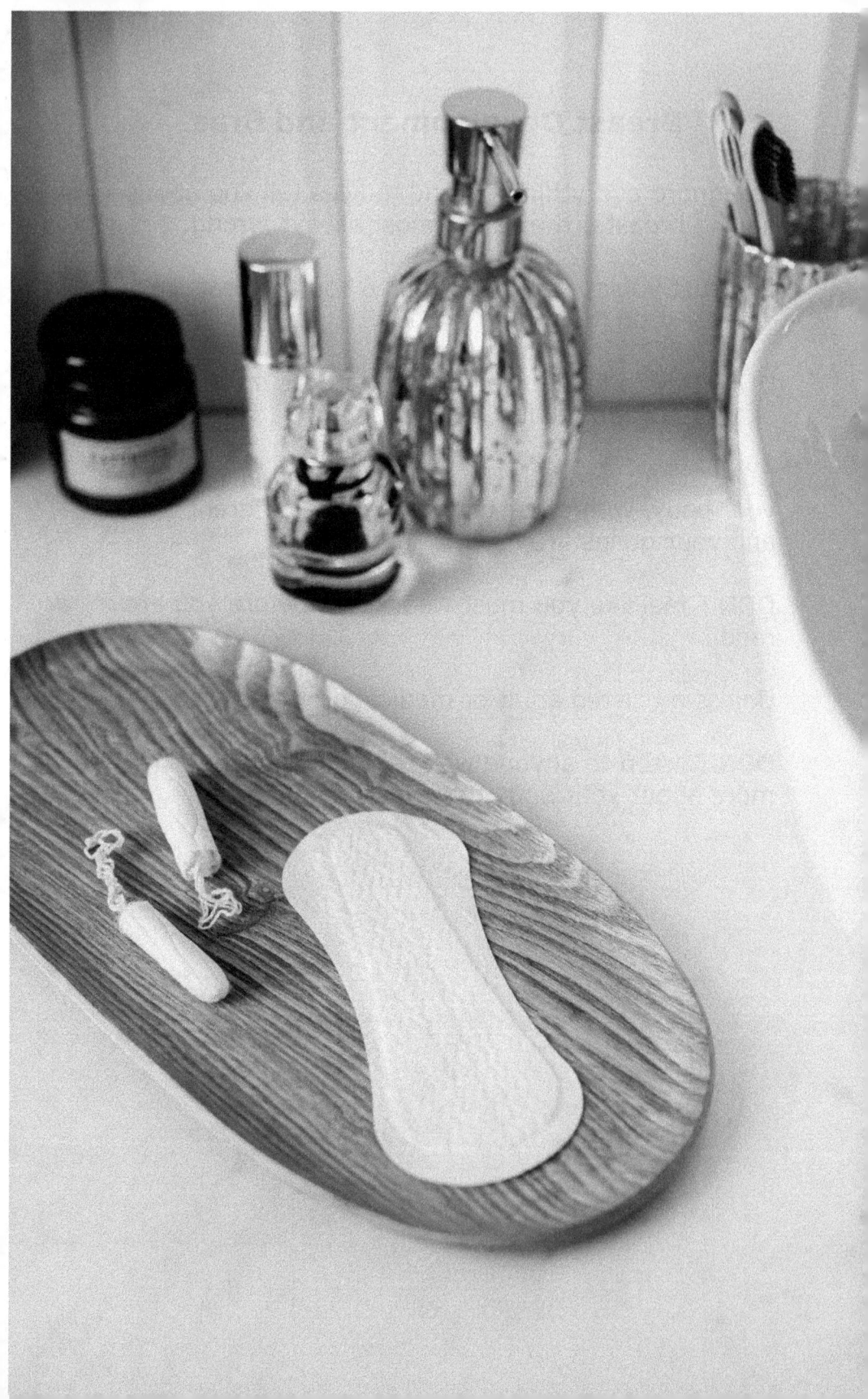

Chapter Three: Menstrual Cycle: Your Period

Menstrual Cycle: Your Period

Menstruation is a period when blood comes out from the girl's vagina. It is the sign when she approaches the end of Puberty. It is the time when you stop looking like a child and become a real girl.

What is commonly called "getting your period" is also known as beginning menstruation. Although this might sound a little scary, it's a normal process that happens every month to women, starting during Puberty and continuing until the age when they can no longer have children.

To understand why this happens, we'll need to do a little anatomy review. Girls are born with a place for babies to hang out and grow until they are ready to come into the world. This place is called the uterus. Not too far from the uterus are two glands called the ovaries. The ovaries' job is to produce estrogen and other hormones and store the eggs that could develop into a baby one day.

Starting in Puberty, about once a month, your ovaries release one of these eggs. The egg travels down a unique egg highway (also known as the fallopian tube) that leads from the ovaries to the uterus. This process takes about three days. If the egg fertilizes (connects with sperm to make the very beginning of a baby), the thickened lining is a nice, cozy spot for the fertilized egg to grow into a baby. If the egg arrives in the uterus and is not fertilized, the uterus doesn't need the extra lining it has built up, so it releases the blood and tissue through the vagina over a few days.

Menstrual Cycle: Your Period

Your first period: how will you know?

When you get your period for the first time, you might feel a small amount of liquid coming out of your vagina. Sometimes it's hard to recognize this feeling initially; it's more likely that you will first see something red or rusty-brown on your underwear.

Your first period can be a little surprising even if you know it's coming (one reason for books like this is so girls won't be surprised), but there is no need to panic! Your period won't start flowing heavily all at once, so you have time to get some supplies. If you're away from home and don't have anything with you, you can ask the school nurse (that is, if you're at school) or the mother or grandmother of one of your friends for sanitary products.

Estrogen and Your Ovaries

Since the beginning of Puberty, your body has been preparing itself for menstruation. It has been releasing a series of hormones necessary for keeping the puberty train running. Now, to be ready for menstruation, your body will need to release two powerful hormones: estrogen (which was mentioned earlier) progesterone. The release of these hormones is how your body knows it's time to pull into the menstruation station.

Menstrual Cycle: Your Period

The Menstrual Cycle

Getting your period is the beginning of a process that takes about 28 days to complete and generally happens once a month.

The time you first see blood until you see blood again the next month is your menstrual cycle. While the average is 28 days, it is normal for you to take more or less time to go through this cycle. During the menstrual cycle, all your reproductive organs work together with your hormones to prepare your body to make a baby someday. It takes a lot of work to grow a human, so your body prepares and practices every month, whether you ever have a baby or not.

Each month, your brain sends a message to your ovaries to start producing estrogen. Your ovaries, the two marble-size organs above your uterus, hold thousands of tiny ova (your eggs), and the production of estrogen is the signal that tells one ovary to release one egg. The process of releasing an egg from the ovary is called ovulation.

How Long Is a Period and When Will I Get Mine?

When you start your period is another bit of secret information that only your body knows. Girls often get their first period around two and a half years from the first sign of breast buds or about six months after they notice vaginal discharge.

Menstrual Cycle: Your Period

However, girls can start their period as young as 9 or as old as 16 whenever you begin is the perfect time for your body.

How long your period will last is also partly determined by your unique body. When you start getting your period, it may be relatively short, around three days or so, and the blood may be just a few pink, light red, or brownish spots in your underwear.

Once your period becomes regular, it can be as short as two days or up to seven. It is also likely that your period will not regularly come in the beginning. Sometimes it can take up to six years for your period to become regular. This train is exciting but can be a bit slow!

How Much Will I Bleed?

Girls can have light periods, heavy periods, or both. Even if a girl has a heavy period with what seems like lots of blood, most girls release only about two tablespoons throughout her period. You may have a little more or a little less. Some girls also get blood clots, which is thicker blood that sometimes comes out in chunks, kind of like jelly, which sounds a little gross, but all of it is normal.

Will Getting My Period Hurt?

Your period is the process of your uterus squeezing out its lining. That squeezing can feel like cramping below your belly button.

Menstrual Cycle: Your Period

Some girls may not feel much of anything when this happens, but it can be uncomfortable for others. After all, your body doesn't use these muscles every day, just a few days a month, and sometimes those muscles get sore. It's like if you went on a long walk up a steep hill, your leg muscles might feel sore the next day. Many of the same things that would make your leg muscles feel better can help your uterine muscles feel better, too: a heating pad, a hot bath, and a little massage.

However, if you feel that you're in a lot of pain before or during your period (like it's hard to get out of bed or get through the school day), be sure to let a trusted adult know. It is something you might want to speak to a doctor about. After all, why should you suffer more than you need to?

My Period and PMS

Your body is so intelligent that it will often give you signals to let you know your period is on the way. These signs aren't the most fun, but they are your body telling you that it is gearing up for some hard and meaningful work. A week or a few days before your period, you may experience breast tenderness, feel a bit moody, feel heavier or bloated around your lower belly, and sometimes have cramps. These symptoms are called premenstrual syndrome (PMS). Lots of girls experience these symptoms, and there are things you can do to reduce them. Eating right is a great way to help your body through PMS.

Menstrual Cycle: Your Period

It takes a lot of nutrients to make the uterine lining every month, so it's essential to eat lots of healthy foods. Foods that contain calcium (yogurt, milk, and so on), iron (green leafy veggies and red meat), fiber (whole grains), and plenty of vitamins (fresh fruits and veggies) will help your body before, during, and after your period. Moving your body with light exercise and movement may also make PMS a little easier for you.

Does Period Blood Smell?

Period blood can have a mild odor, but no one can smell it through your clothes. No one will know you have your period unless you tell them. Washing daily and wearing clean underwear helps keep down smelly bacteria. It is true during your period as well. Changing your pad or tampon regularly can also help you feel fresh during your period.

Tracking Your Period

Another way to know when to expect your period is to track it. Your menstrual cycle begins on the first day of your period (the first day you see blood) in one month and runs to the first day of your period in the next month. The average cycle is 28 days, but it can be as long as 45 or as short as 21.

On the first day of your period, draw a small heart on that day on your calendar. Draw a heart for each day of your period. After your period is over, count the days until your next period begins. Begin counting from your first heart until your next period.

Menstrual Cycle: Your Period

That number of days is your cycle. Your cycle will take time to get regular, so the numbers may not be the same for a while. You can also use cool apps and websites to help you track your period, so you know when it's coming.

No matter when you get your first period, give yourself a high five when it arrives. Your body did some fantastic work to get it here!

Personal Period Care

Let's talk about care and hygiene during "that time of the month." Soon you will have all you need to know about pads, tampons, and more so that you can navigate menstruation with ease.

Pads, Tampons, and More

You will have your period for many days of your life while you are out there becoming who you want to be, and your period should not be something that holds you back. Thankfully, there are various products to choose from, so you don't have to skip any activities when you have your period. Many stores have an entire aisle of what they call feminine hygiene products or menstrual care products—products made just for period care. The goal is for you to be comfortable, clean, and worry-free during menstruation.

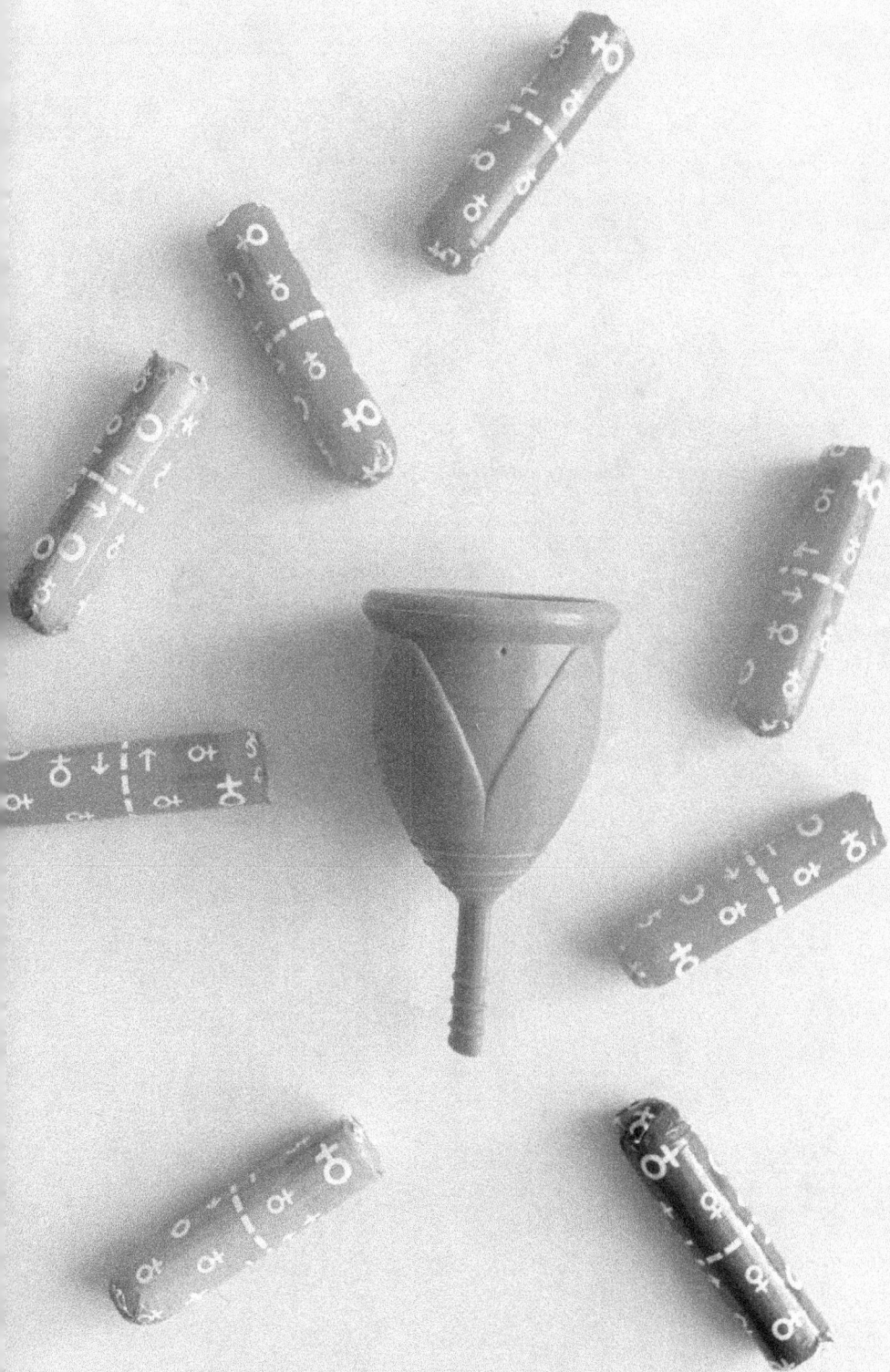

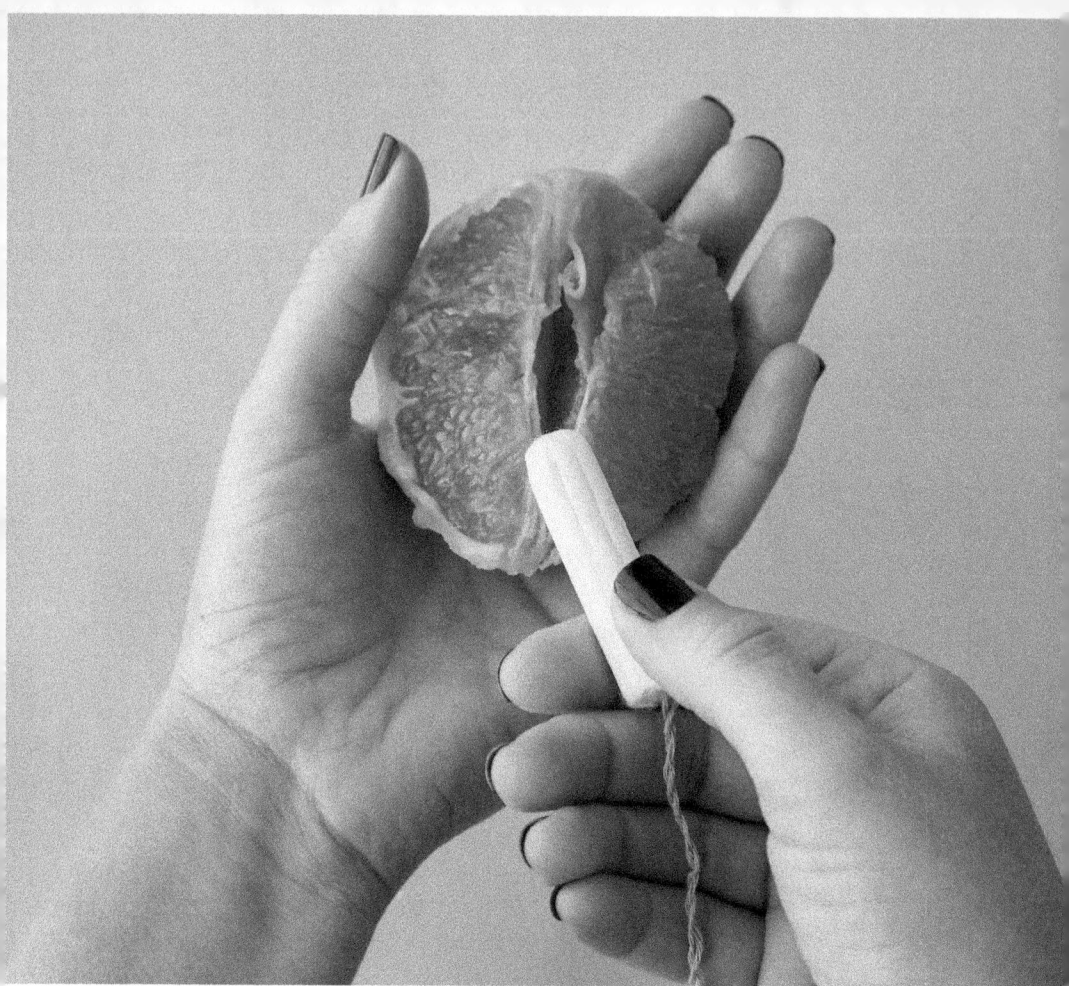

Menstrual Cycle: Your Period

Pads and tampons are the two most common products girls use to take care of their menstrual bleeding. Pads are absorbent liners worn in your underwear to soak up the blood coming out of your vagina. Tampons are cotton plugs that you insert into your vagina to catch the blood before leaving your body. You don't have to choose just one type of product. You may use different products depending on the situation. Pads are easy and are the most common product to start with when you first get your period. Tampons require a bit more learning, and it takes time to get comfortable using them.

What you use depends on your activity and your personal preference. It's like deciding what kind of backpack or purse you like to carry. Not everyone likes the same things. For example, wearing a leotard or bathing suit may require you to figure out how to use a tampon quicker than your best friend, who doesn't do gymnastics or swim. A vacation for a week at the beach may change your mind about trying tampons.

Another feminine hygiene product is a menstrual cup. It is a reusable device that you insert into your vagina to collect the blood rather than absorb it. You then remove the cup from your vagina periodically throughout the day, empty it, rinse and clean it, and reinsert it back into the vagina. It's much more environmentally friendly than pads or tampons, but it's often not used by beginners. Inserting a menstrual cup requires you to be very comfortable with your body.

Menstrual Cycle: Your Period

Reusable, washable underwear that absorbs the blood from your period is another excellent option. These can replace pads or tampons or menstrual cups or even be worn along with them for extra protection. There are many brands and styles to choose from, such as Thinx, Knix, and Ruby Love.

How to Shop for Supplies

Most drugstores, grocery stores, and any place that sells body care products will have tampons and pads. Menstrual cups can be a little harder to find and a bit more expensive at first.

You may need to go to a health food or natural products store to get them. Unlike pads and tampons that need to be replaced regularly, menstrual cups can last for years with good care.

Pads and tampons come in different sizes, and absorbencies (how much fluid they can soak up) for heavy, regular, and light flows. Of course, companies also make all sorts of other styles, hoping that you will buy more.

Getting Rid of Used Pads

Pads are disposable but cannot be flushed down the toilet. They can clog up the plumbing! To properly dispose of your pad, roll it up with the sticky part on the outside. Once it is tightly rolled, wrap the pad in toilet paper and throw it in the trash. If you have a pet dog, be sure to put the used pad in a trash can the dog cannot get into.

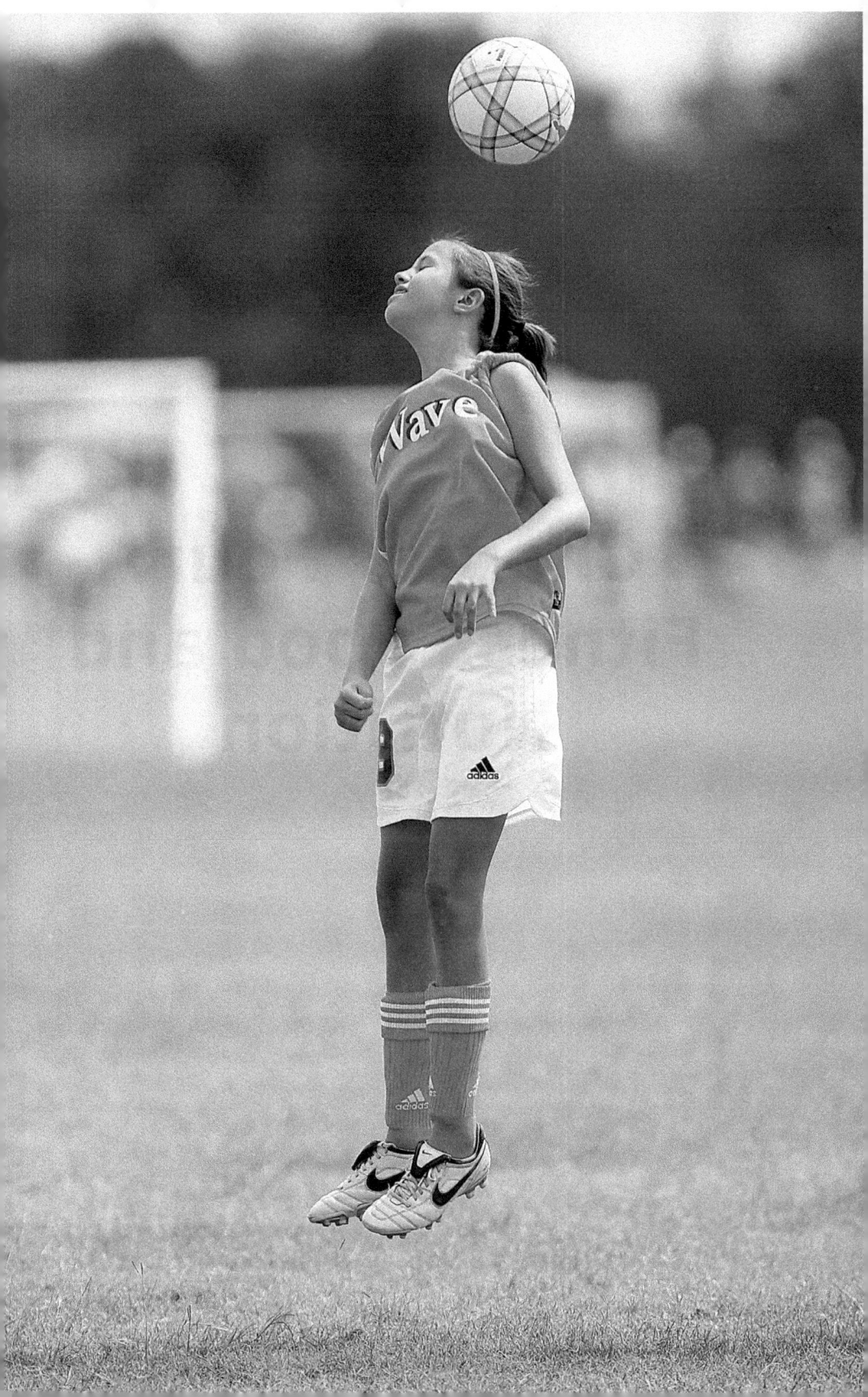

Chapter Four: Fitness Food and Nutrition

Nutrition and health go hand in hand. Taking care of your body means feeding yourself foods that nourish you. Your body is like a machine, and the fuel we put in it matters. Fueling your body with foods that nourish you will keep your body feeling strong and healthy.

There are many challenges to healthy eating. All around us, there are restaurants, ice cream parlors, and treats. Often you may notice that it's challenging to make healthy choices if you are on the go. Making your nutrition a priority means that you have to plan your meals and be prepared. We understand that you are not always preparing your food at home or school, so do your best to make wise choices with what you are offered.

Your body is on a once-in-a-lifetime journey of growing and changing. To ride on a healthy puberty train, you will need wholesome and nutritious food. Often when we hear the word nutrition, we think of being forced to eat the yuckiest foods. Luckily, nutrition doesn't mean suffering through endless meals with peas or whatever you don't like. Eating nutritious food can mean enjoying delicious food as well. Good for you can taste good, too.

Getting proper nutrition can not only affect how you grow during Puberty; it can also affect how early or late you start Puberty. Not getting enough healthy food can keep your body from launching the necessary hormones to begin Puberty.

Fitness Food and Nutrition

And overeating unhealthy food can cause your body to begin puberty changes sooner than it is supposed to. Since getting nutritious food is such a big deal for growing bodies like yours, let's talk about how to fuel your body.

A Rainbow of Flavors

One easy way to make sure you're getting lots of the healthy food you need to help your body handle Puberty like a champ is to eat a rainbow. Okay, just kidding—you are not going to eat an actual rainbow. That would be quite a feat!

Eating the rainbow means eating natural foods that make up the rainbow's colors, making it easier to get the vitamins and minerals your body needs to develop through Puberty. Here are the yummy colors you will want to see on your plate and how they will help your body grow.

RED: apples, cherries, red cabbage, strawberries, tomatoes, watermelon. Red foods can help you develop a sharp memory and a healthy heart.

ORANGE/YELLOW: butternut squash, cantaloupes, carrots, mangos, oranges, pineapples, potatoes, sweet potatoes, yellow peppers. Eating from the yellow part of the rainbow means getting the vitamins you need to have healthy eyes, heart, and immune systems.

Fitness Food and Nutrition

GREEN: Green apples, avocados, grapes, Kale, Spinach, zucchini.

PURPLE/BLUE: beets, blackberries, blueberries, dark beans, eggplant, figs. Purple and blue foods will boost your memory and help your body stay strong as you age.

WHITE: ginger, mushrooms, onions.
White foods will help keep your heart pumping strong and healthy.

But," you say, "what if I make a rainbow of orange cheddar potato chips, strawberry fruit snacks, and green apple gummy bears? Can that count as eating the rainbow?" Well, while those colors are found in the rainbow, you will probably get a bellyache and a trip to the dentist for cavities faster than you will get the nutrition you need for your body. Nope, rainbow-colored junk food will not help the puberty train have a smooth ride. And foods that are high in sugar, fats, and salts can cause health problems as you get older.

It does not mean you can never eat chips, candy, or cake. They are fine in moderation, though they should never replace fruits, vegetables, and grains on the breakfast, lunch, or dinner table. Fresh, natural food that is close to its original form will always be healthier for you. It means trying to avoid processed foods.

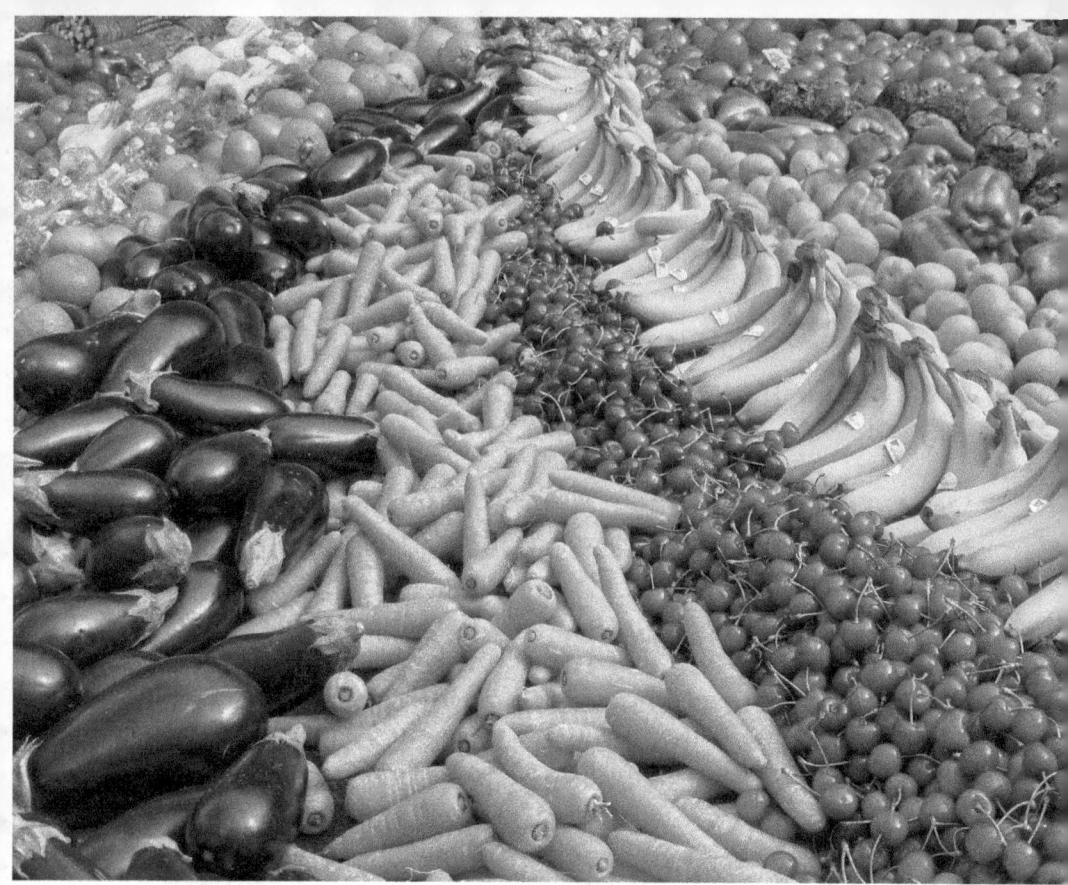

Fitness Food and Nutrition

The best way to know if a food is processed is to look at its packaging. Foods that come in boxes and cans or contain powders, syrups, or other flavorings are usually processed. Processed foods often have had lots of sugar, salt, and fats added to them, while many of the nutrients have been stripped away. It is better to look for fresh food choices whenever you can. For example, fresh peach is going to give you more nutrition than canned peaches in sugary syrup.

Your body will need a few other nutrients to keep it in tip-top shape. Foods with protein—like meat, fish, beans, and cheese—will help you develop healthy muscles. You will also need foods with iron in them for energy, zinc to help your body fight illness, and folates to help your body soak up needed minerals.

Be a healthy food helper!

Ask the grown-up who does the grocery shopping if you can tag along and help them pick out delicious rainbow-colored fresh food. Tell them it will be good for your taste buds, as well as your rapidly growing body.

Start Your Day the Right Way

One of the best gifts you can give your brilliant body is breakfast. Eating breakfast each day is like saying, "Good morning, body! Glad to see you today!" Breakfast is perhaps the most important meal of the day. It gives your body the energy it needs to start running all those complicated functions that keep you alive.

Fitness Food and Nutrition

It also helps you not feel cranky and tired in the afternoon. Great breakfast ideas include oatmeal, fruit smoothies, eggs and toast, and bananas and peanut butter.

Allergies, Veggies Only, and Other Special Food Needs

People have different nutritional needs, and their bodies react differently to food. Some people can't eat gluten (wheat products), and others have severe food allergies. Caring for our bodies sometimes means taking care of our unique food needs. Food allergies—when foods cause an adverse physical reaction in our bodies if we eat them (like itching, swelling, or other dangerous reactions)—are a common issue for many young people. Up to three million people in the United States are allergic to some food. Unfortunately, just because food isn't suitable for your body doesn't mean it won't taste good. And this is where you can find yourself in trouble. Never eat foods you know you are allergic to, no matter how tasty they may look.

Hormone increases, and stress during Puberty can make allergies worse. So continue to eat healthily and be sure to stay away from foods that will trigger a reaction—your body will thank you!

Vegetarians are people who do not eat meat. People become vegetarian for many reasons, including religion and caring about animals.

Fitness Food and Nutrition

If you are a vegetarian or are considering becoming one, you'll need to figure out ways to get all the nutrition you need from other foods. You will need extra protein and vitamins (like B12) that are primarily found in meat products. Talk with an adult and a doctor who can help make sure you are getting what your body needs to grow.

Move Your Body

One of the best ways to help your body is to move it! Exercise—getting up and moving around—is a beautiful way to support your ever-changing body. Now that doesn't mean you need to do 300 jumping jacks and run 12 laps around the gym unless you like jumping jacks and running! But you should find ways to move your body that make you happy and sweaty.

Do you love dancing?

Ask your parent or a teacher to help you find a dance class. Or you can make up dance routines at home. Do you love sports? Join your school's basketball, softball, or soccer team (or whatever sport you like). You could even get your friends in the neighborhood to play on weekends. There are endless possibilities for how to move your body. The important thing is that you get moving.

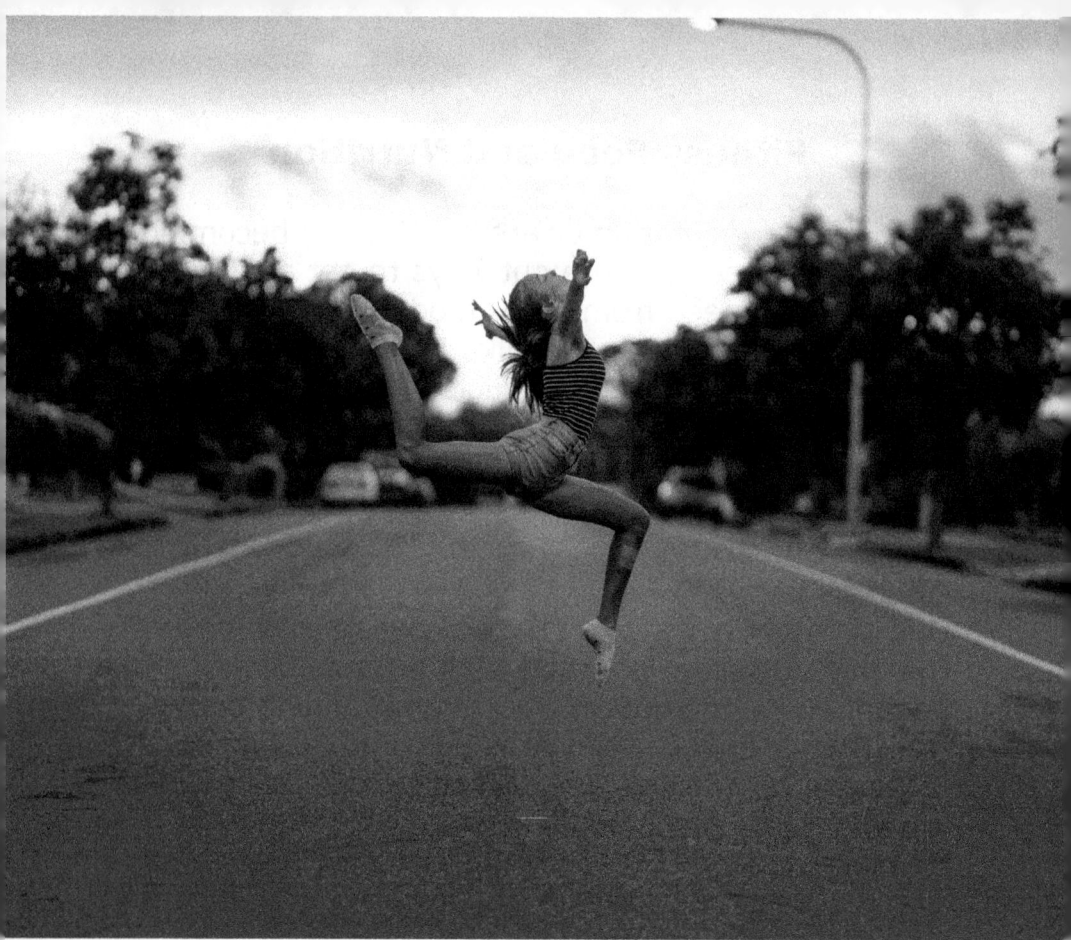

Fitness Food and Nutrition

Not all families are active or focus on their physical health. You may feel empowered by reading this to do things that benefit your health and then become a role model for your family and make exercise a family activity. The change can start with you.

What Do I Get Out of Exercise?

Exercise benefits your body and mind; everyone should get at least 60 minutes of exercise a day. The exercise should make your heart and lungs work harder and move faster.

It doesn't have to be an organized sport or an expensive class at the nearby fitness center. You can achieve your exercise goal with a gym class at school, walking around your block, meeting friends for a bike ride, or even just cranking up the music and dancing in your room.

It's impressive that exercise:

Improves your mood

It helps you sleep better

It makes your muscles and bones stronger

Encourages other healthy habits

It allows you to meet new people

Improves your confidence

Fitness Food and Nutrition

How Much Do I Need to Move?

Most doctors suggest that you move at least one hour a day. If you are doing stuff you love to do, it will be easy to get to an hour. Sixty minutes may sound like a lot of activity if you are currently inactive. You don't have to reach this goal overnight. Like any goal you want to achieve, it will take effort and perseverance. Set small, realistic goals and build up slowly. Start with a goal of a 10-minute walk around the block. As this becomes easier, you can increase the amount of time and effort until you reach your goal.

But remember, even a little exercise is better than none. If getting out and moving is hard because you haven't done it for a while, start small and work your way up. Try going for a walk with a friend for 20 minutes, or ask a neighbor if you can walk their dog. The more often you practice moving your body, the easier it is to do. If you have a disability that makes exercise difficult, try to think of exercises that work for your body and feel fun. Do them for as long as you can. Movement can look different for different bodies.

And for inspiration, here are a few fun Move Your Body games to play at home!

1.Headstands: Strengthen your stomach muscles and get that blood to your brain by practicing a headstand.

Fitness Food and Nutrition

2.Jump rope: Get your heartbeat going with this fun exercise. Go outside and get friends to join you.

3.Wheelbarrow, crab, and bear-walk races: You and your partner (you will need one) will build arm, leg, and stomach strength with these games.

4.Animal races: Bunnyhop, frog leap, and quack around like a duck to see who can get the farthest.

5.Obstacle course: Create an obstacle course indoors with pillows, stuffed animals, and toys (just be sure to ask an adult before you start moving furniture). Or you can map a course outside with sidewalk chalk.

Moving Your Body Safely

Our bodies are sturdy, but they are also delicate and need some care before we start moving them around. Warming up and cooling down is especially important if you play on a sports team or dance in a company; dancers and athletes may get injuries more often because of the stress both activities can put on muscles and bones.

It is essential to warm your muscles up before you begin exercising. Warm-ups can include stretches, light walking, slow swimming, and any other easy movement that helps your muscles prepare for a workout.

Fitness Food and Nutrition

You will also want to cool down after you exercise. Cool-downs help your body slowly return to a state of rest. Suddenly stopping during exercise can shock your muscles and cause soreness or more severe injuries. You will want to slow down your movement or return to stretching until you feel your heartbeat slows down. Once your heart is beating more slowly, and your breathing has slowed down, you can safely rest your body.

Stay Hydrated

Guess what your body absolutely must have to live— water! Water is the most magical fluid in the world. Did you know that your body is made up of mostly water? So, of course, your body is magic! Water is the best drink you can give your body, helping it continue to feel good and work properly.

Exactly how much water you should drink each day is up for some debate. But what we know for sure is that you should drink more water than any other drink. Sodas and juices often have tons of sugar and salt in them, which don't help your body work well when you drink too much of them. You should drink one to two glasses of water before you start exercising, a glass during your exercise, and at least one glass afterward. If you wait to drink water until you are thirsty, your body is already low on the water it needs.

Fitness Food and Nutrition

Sleep

Whether you still love a bedtime story or you drift off to dreamland right when your head hits the pillow, one thing is for sure: Your body needs sleep and lots of it if you are going to stay healthy and happy during (and after) Puberty. Your body is growing faster than at almost any other point in your life. New hormones are being made to help your body begin all sorts of new functions, and these significant changes take an enormous amount of energy. How do you make sure your body has what it needs to succeed at growing your great body? One essential way is by making sure you get enough sleep.

How Much Sleep Is Enough?

Girls between the ages of 8 and 11 should be getting between 9 and 11 hours of sleep per night. To take good care of your body, you may need to miss the late shows on TV.

Why Do I Need So Much Sleep?

As your body prepares for Puberty, you may notice yourself being sleepier than usual or having a more challenging time waking up in the morning. Needing more sleep is a normal part of Puberty. Remember, your body is taking on some big new tasks like growth spurts (most bone growth happens while you sleep), producing hormones, and growing whole new body parts like breasts. That is a tremendous amount of work your body is doing, and it needs the energy to do it.

Fitness Food and Nutrition

If you don't get the sleep you need, it can affect your memory, ability to learn and understand, and mood. You simply don't want to be a cranky, exhausted, sleepy person for your spelling test. One of the best ways to make sure your brain and body are working in their best condition is to give them lots of good sleep.

What Won't Help

While nutrition, exercise, and sleep will help you keep the puberty train moving, three things will leave you and your body stuck on the tracks—so say no.

Smoking

Cigarettes were created to help companies earn tons of money from making you think smoking is cool. Companies get wealthy convincing young people to start smoking early because they know cigarettes are addictive (once you start, it is hard for your body to stop).

Here's what you need to remember:

First, you are too smart to let some sneaky company take advantage of you for years. And second, just about everybody knows that cigarettes don't just make you cough and make your clothes and hair and breath smell gross—they can be deadly. Cigarettes cause cancer, lung disease, and all sorts of other life-threatening conditions. Don't let slimy companies cheat you out of your health or your money. Don't smoke!

Fitness Food and Nutrition

Alcohol and Drugs

Billboards, commercials, and magazines are constantly talking about alcohol. TV shows and news programs are constantly talking about drugs. Why? For the same reason, cigarette companies talk about cigarettes. Companies make lots of money when people buy and drink alcohol, and drug dealers make lots of money when people buy and use drugs.

Here's the deal:

Drugs and alcohol are super dangerous for young people. Yes, they can be super dangerous for adults, too. But your body is changing and developing in serious ways during Puberty.

Alcohol and drugs can hurt that process and cause you problems into adulthood. Both alcohol and drugs (including marijuana) can cause brain damage and hurt your kidneys, liver, and heart as they grow. Simply put, drugs and alcohol can cause you lots of harm.

Some kids try to make drinking, doing drugs, and smoking seem like the cool thing to do. Often, kids do this because they don't feel good about themselves or have problems in their lives they don't know how to deal with. Feel free to seek advice from an adult you trust and talk about these feelings and issues.

Fitness Food and Nutrition

It's okay to ask for help. You don't have to go through any of the hard stuff alone. Growing up can feel overwhelming sometimes, but you have all the power and smarts inside you that you need to grow into a fantastic and brave young person—and you don't need drugs and alcohol to do it.

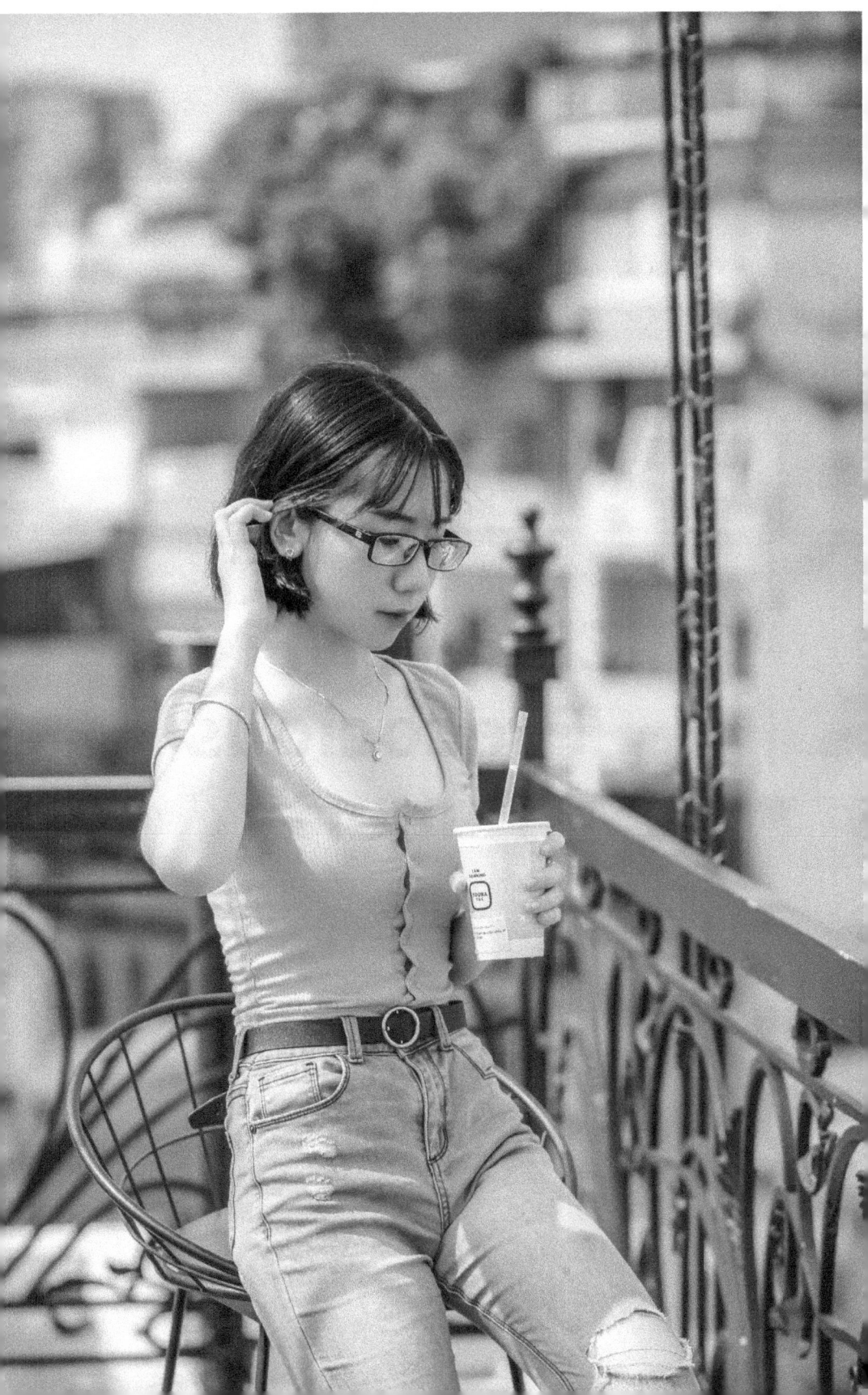

Chapter Five: Precocious Puberty

Precocious Puberty

What does this mean?

Well, we don't all go through Puberty at the same time. Some girls start to show puberty signs at a very young age, even as young as 5. But usually precocious Puberty or early Puberty in girls happens between the ages of 7 to 10. For example, a girl may have her first period below the age of 8 years. That is a sign of precocious Puberty.

It usually starts with the breasts start to grow and feel sore, underarms hair starts to grow, a growth spurt where the girl gets taller quickly, body odor, and sometimes pimples.

Typically, these signs will happen for a couple of years before the girl gets her first period. It can be a tough time for young girls, both physically and emotionally. If this happens to you, don't worry, you are normal, and all your friends will eventually go through Puberty as well.

Precocious Puberty can either be central or peripheral. Central precocious Puberty occurs when the brain abnormally secretes gonadotropins at a younger age. The pituitary gland releases gonadotropin hormones signaling gonads in girls' ovaries. Its cause is, however, not clear.

Peripheral precocious Puberty occurs when estrogen hormone is produced early in other body parts. In girls, it may also occur as a result of ovarian cysts and tumors.

Precocious Puberty

Precocious Puberty Symptoms

The signs and symptoms of precocious Puberty and Puberty are the same; the only difference is timing. In girls, the first visible sign is breast development. Menstrual flow may also come earlier than expected.

Causes of Early Puberty

In most cases, experts do not usually know what causes central precocious Puberty. A medical problem like brain injury from surgery may trigger precocious Puberty in girls. Other complications like brain inflammations and tumors may also be a significant cause.

Precocious Puberty risk factors

Gender: girls are more likely to experience precocious Puberty than boys

Genetics: genetic mutations may lead to precocious Puberty as they trigger the release of sexual hormones. A child may experience early Puberty because a sibling or parent has similar genetic conditions.

Race: African American girls are believed to start Puberty a year earlier on average than white girls.

Treatment of Precocious Puberty...

Precocious Puberty

If you sense your child is experiencing early Puberty, it is advisable to consult a specialist to examine your child. It is usual for the specialist to run tests, for instance, a blood test to check for hormone levels or an MRI scan that usually detects any possibility of a tumor.

It is advised to treat any underlying conditions that may be the primary cause of precocious Puberty. Seek medications to delay sexual development and reduce hormonal levels.

The type of treatment doctors suggests usually depends on the exact cause of your child's early Puberty.

Watchful waiting:

In this case, a doctor may suggest watching your child for a few months as there may be no cause. GnRH analogue therapy: This is a medication that a doctor advises that your child gets once a month in a shot only if your child has precocious Puberty and no other conditions. As your child takes the medication, it halts development until they reach the average puberty age.

Histrelin mplant (Vantas):

An implant that a doctor puts under the inside part of the upper arm's skin. It usually delays development and requires minor surgery to install the implant. It lasts a year and hence does not require any monthly shots.

Precocious Puberty

How Precocious Puberty affects kids

Short height

Precocious Puberty usually makes kids not reach their full adult height potential mainly because growth in height stops when Puberty ends. Their bone growth stops at an earlier age than normal. They may initially appear taller than their peers but eventually may end up shorter.

Social problems

Precocious Puberty may also pose emotional and social problems to the kids affected. For example, girls may feel shy and embarrassed when their breasts develop much earlier than their peers. Other children may also tease them and become emotionally draining incredibly for girls.
To fit in, they may opt to hang out with older kids who may introduce them to bad, unhealthy habits like alcohol abuse.

Poor body image and low self-esteem

Early breast development and sprouting body hair may make girls develop low self-esteem. It is because they become self-conscious as they feel different than their peers. Girls may get sexual attention because of their body changes, and this can make them feel quite uncomfortable.

Precocious Puberty

Anxiety and Depression

Early Puberty may not give a child enough time to learn the coping skills to deal with depression and anxiety. Flood of hormones, especially oestrone in girls, may make depression more likely.

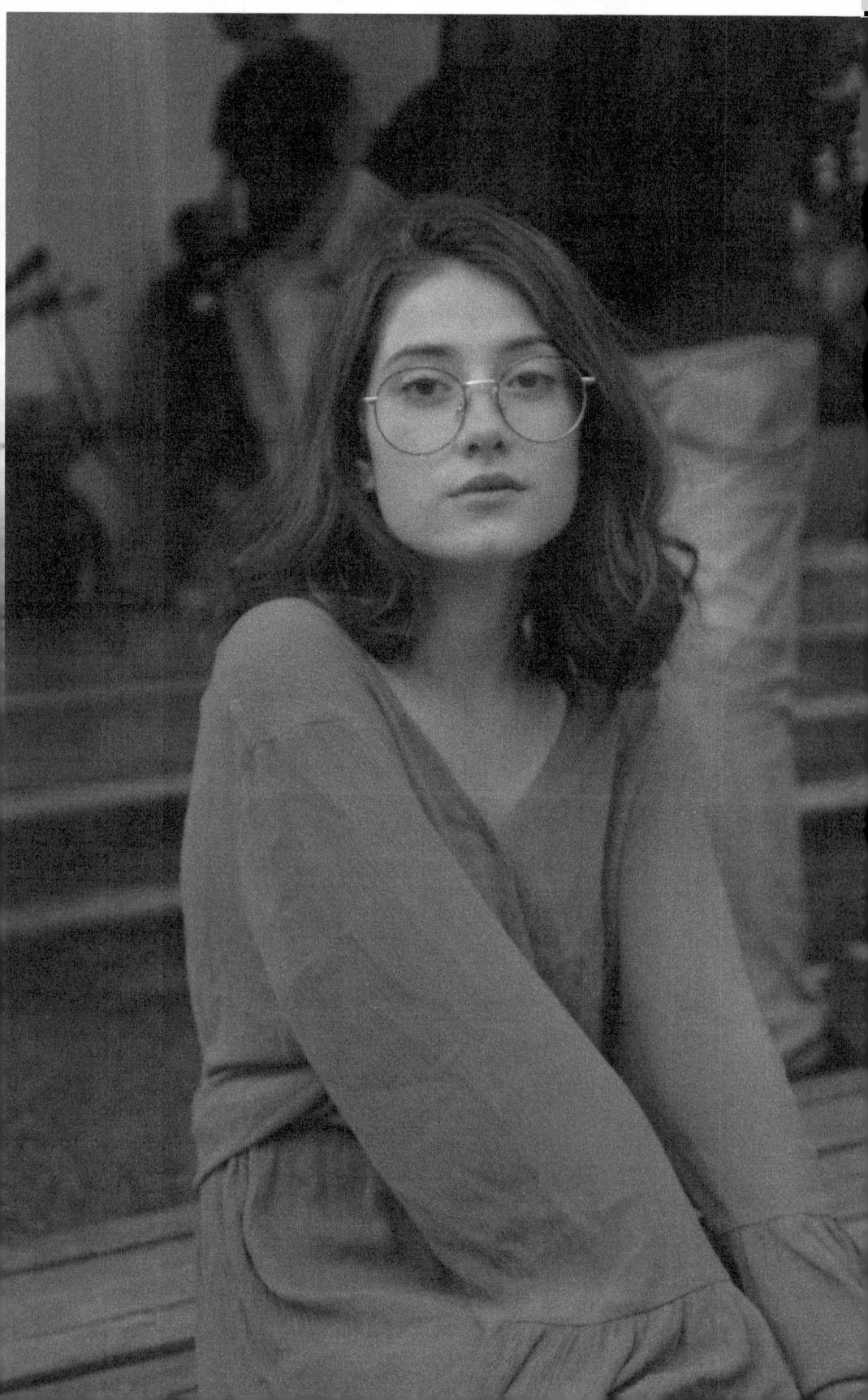

Chapter Six: Puberty and Emotions

Puberty and Emotions

While Puberty is most definitely a train ride, on occasion, it can feel more like a roller coaster with some high hills and steep drops along the way. Have you ever stormed off to your room because your mom said something you didn't like? Do you sometimes feel like your feelings are all over the place? A large part of what you're experiencing results from something we've talked about throughout this book. Any guesses? Go ahead; I bet you know. Yes! Good old hormones. Your body is producing new chemicals to help you grow ever so slowly into an adult. These hormones affect many of your body's functions, but they also affect your emotions.

Why Are My Feelings So Intense?

Humans feel things: Joy, sadness, anger, frustration, confusion, worry, wonder, excitement, fear, and a thousand other feelings we might not even have words for yet! Strong emotions are part of being human. As your body adjusts to the new hormones you are producing, you may notice that your feelings feel more prominent than they have ever felt before. These feelings may make you more sensitive than usual. Some days you may feel like crying for no apparent reason. At other moments you may feel super angry about something that used just to irritate you a little. All of this is normal and okay.

Puberty and Emotions

Of course, your changing feelings can be awkward and intense. You may also be experiencing new emotions like jealousy or even romantic feelings toward a friend or classmate. You may feel misunderstood or proud. You may have questions about yourself and the world that you never had before. The more experiences you have, the more feelings are possible.

No matter what feelings you may experience during this time, it is essential to know that you are important, intelligent, and capable. You are good enough, no matter what feelings show up. Always remember, feelings do not last forever. They change very quickly. Take a deep breath and stay on the train. It's just part of the ride. Uncertainty about your feelings might keep you from seeing that, and that's normal! The more you understand your feelings and emotions, the less confused you will feel as you grow and change. You may not realize it, but you already have everything you need inside you to handle these changes. But specific tools and tricks can make it much easier—and that's where this book comes in.

There are at least two reasons for mood swings. The first is the hormonal changes that are going on in your body. Yes, that pesky estrogen strikes again! The second has to do with your changing place in the world. Puberty is the bridge between being a girl and being a woman, and sometimes you might feel like you don't belong in either place.

Puberty and Emotions

You aren't a kid anymore, but sometimes you feel like one inside and still want to do kid things. On the other hand, you aren't ready for the responsibilities that come with being an adult, even though you may feel like you want and need more independence. Some days you might feel out of place and like no one understands what you're going through. No wonder you might be a little (or a lot) cranky! Talking about your feelings can help keep those emotions in check. Don't worry if it is hard for you to open up—everyone feels this way sometimes. A trusted adult will understand if it is difficult for you to get the words out.

Your feelings are a lot like waves. Sometimes feelings can be immense, choppy, scary waves. Sometimes you're happy because the waves are small and smooth—of course, this is when it's easier to navigate the boat.

The mood swings during Puberty happen for many reasons. Not only are you dealing with a flood of hormones, you are also trying to handle the anxiety that comes along with the process itself.

You are probably a little concerned about how you are developing and what your friends and family might think. Anxiety can make everything seem so much worse than it is, leading to significant mood swings.

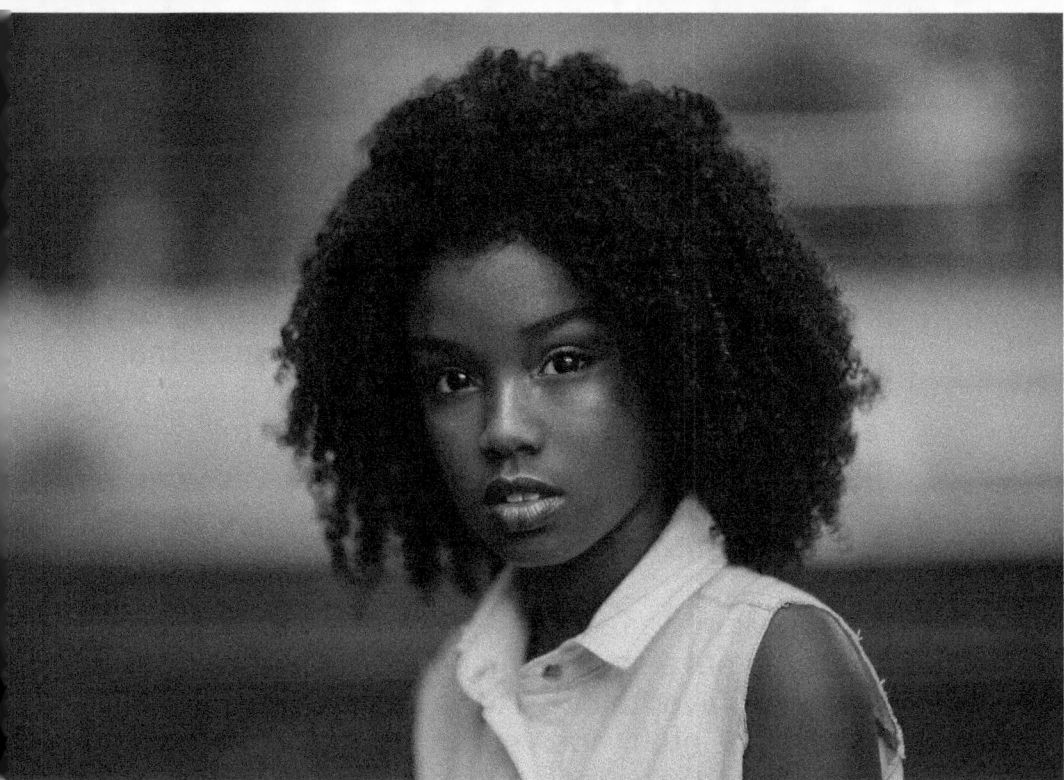

Puberty and Emotions

The best way to combat mood swings is to understand them. You know they are coming from the changing hormones, and there is little you can do about that. So be kind to yourself! Recognize that you are going to have mood swings. It's a fact. You can, however, help yourself by doing the following things:

Expressing Emotions

It's important to feel like you can be yourself, even when you have strong emotions. If you didn't get to wear your favorite outfit for picture day, you might feel disappointed, and your mood may shift from happy to sad. You may be less talkative when you're upset or want to be left alone. When this happens, your friends may comment or ask what's wrong. It means that you've expressed yourself in a way that tells others a story about how you feel.

Emotional expression is the way you choose to show your feelings. There is no wrong or right way to do this, but some ways of expressing your emotions are healthier than others.

Many young ladies enjoy their teenage years and do not necessarily desire to change. However, things change during Puberty, and there is nothing anyone can do to stop it. Teenagers do not have to be fearful of Puberty, growth, and changes.

Puberty and Emotions

How Can I Manage My Mood?

You may feel like your emotions are running the show and just dragging you along. But you don't have to hang on to the caboose on this train ride.

There are things you can do to help manage your emotions during Puberty. But it's important to know how to deal with them in a way that leaves you feeling better, not worse.

There are no right or wrong emotions to have, but some not-so-nice ways of expressing yourself, such as fighting or yelling. I'm going to share some tips and tricks for handling your emotions. They can help you feel better when you feel bad and can help you express yourself in the most healthily way. When you're able to express yourself more calmly or kindly, your friendships and relationships with others are better, too. Let's talk about some of these techniques:

Meditation

Sitting quietly for a few minutes each day and letting your mind practice being quiet can also help your moods. This practice is called meditation, and it is an excellent tool for helping you cope when your emotions feel out of control. Meditation teaches you how to sit with your feelings until they leave. Feelings can be like houseguests who don't stay very long. They usually don't plan on moving in.

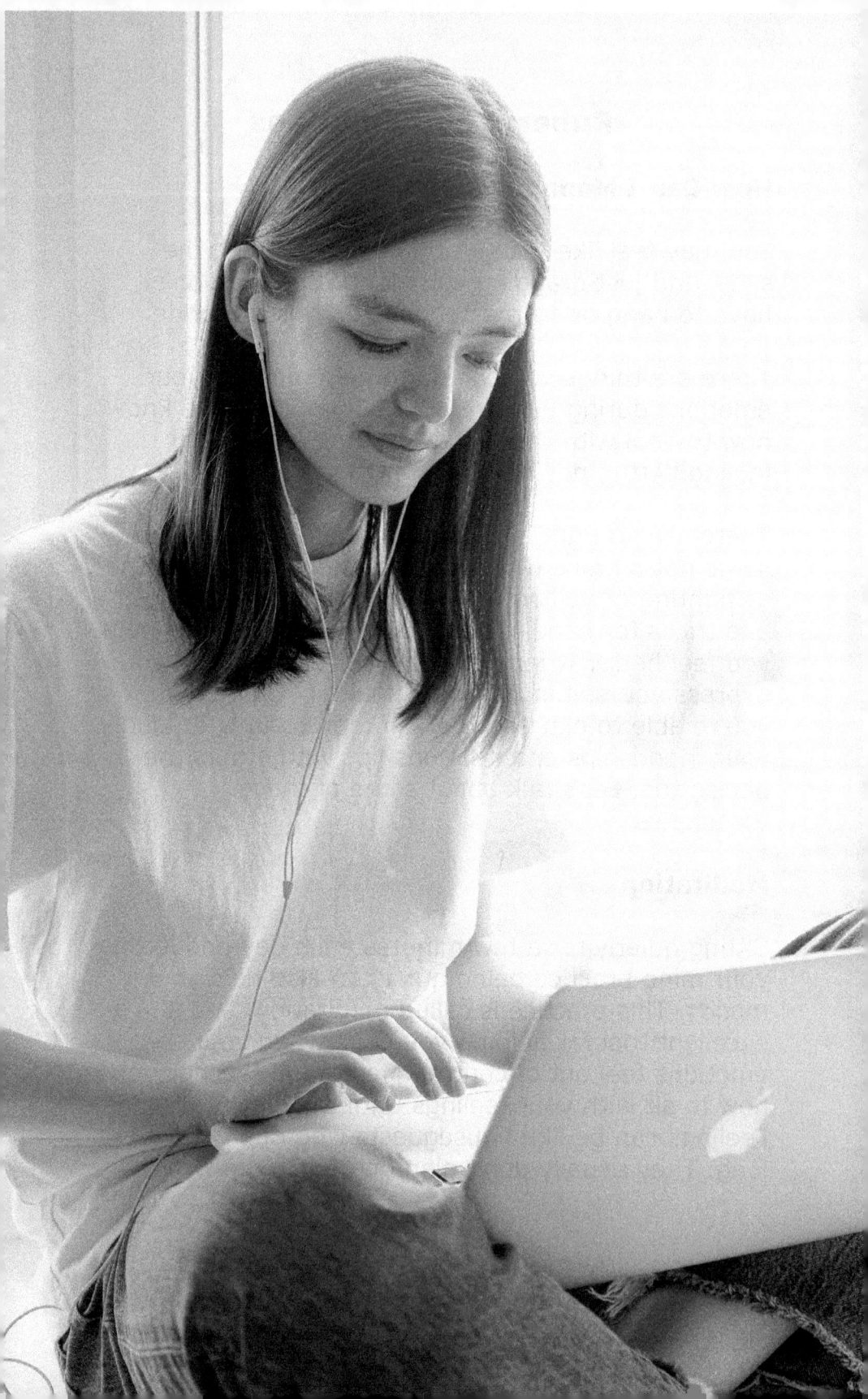

Puberty and Emotions

Back to the Big Three

Eating healthy food will make your moods easier to handle. A sure way to feel cranky and frustrated is to let yourself get too hungry or to eat food that doesn't feel good inside your body. When you don't eat, your body gets slow and sluggish. As you lose the energy, your mood can also begin to go down. There is nothing worse than being hungry and angry at the same time—or what we call hangry. Don't be hangry. Eat three healthy meals and small healthy snacks throughout the day.

Exercise releases chemicals in your brain that make you feel good—feeling frustrated? Take a walk around the block. Are you feeling sad? Try swimming some laps in your local pool or throw on some music and dance the happiness back into your body.

And don't forget about sleep. Your mind and body need time to recharge. Sleep is like food for your brain. Your mind will get hangry if it doesn't get what it needs, which is 9 to 11 hours of sleep each night.

Talk or Write It Out

Having all these solid and new emotions can feel confusing. One way to lessen the confusion is to get the ideas out of your head. Talking about your feelings with a trusted adult who cares about you, believes in you, and wants the best for you is a beautiful way to move through challenging emotions without feeling like you are alone.

Puberty and Emotions

Find an adult who is a good listener and can talk to you about what you're feeling. They went through Puberty too and may have the right words to help you.

Another great way to let those feelings out is to write in a journal. Write down your fears, joys, and successes. Write when someone makes you boiling with anger or when a friend hurts you. Write when your outfit is fabulous or when you think your classmates are judging you. Writing is an easy but effective way to let out your feelings in a safe place.

Maybe you can share your journal with someone you trust, or maybe it is just for you. Either way, writing can help you sort through the roller-coaster ride of feelings in a healthy way.

Breathe deeply.

Thankfully, breathing is so automatic that we never have to think about doing it! Sometimes, though, it can be helpful to notice your breaths and practice breathing deeply and slowly. Deep breathing lowers your feelings of anxiety and can make you feel calm and even sleepy. There are a couple of fun ways to practice deep breathing:

Take a big, deep breath in for four seconds, hold it for another four seconds, and then slowly exhale for another four seconds. Repeat this a few times until you feel calm.

Puberty and Emotions

Place your favorite stuffed animal or blanket on your tummy and watch it go up and down as you take big, deep breaths in and out.

Relax those muscles.

When we feel stressed out, our brain sends a message to the body to prepare for danger. It causes our muscles to feel tense. If this happens a lot, it can cause pain throughout your body, such as headaches or sore shoulders. To relax your tight muscles, try this:

Take a big breath in, and squeeze those muscles until they feel tight or tense. Then relax and slowly let go of the pressure, breathing out as you go. For example, try putting both of your fists into a tight ball and holding it for a few seconds before letting go slowly. When you let go, breathe out slowly and count to 10. It's helpful to relax your shoulders and jaw as you release, too.

Find your safe space.

Close your eyes and let your imagination take over! I want you to imagine and describe your happiest or safest place. It can be a real place you've been, or you can make it up and decorate it how you want. Be sure to include:

Puberty and Emotions

The sights, including the color of the walls or sky

The smells

The temperature

The sounds

What you're wearing

Who is or isn't there

Be as detailed and creative as you want—you may even want to imagine what superpowers you have! Want to relax even more? Do this activity along with deep breathing.

Practice mindfulness.

Do you ever feel that your thoughts and feelings are like a loud storm in your head? Sometimes you may wish you could quiet that storm. You can, and here's how:

Try to imagine your thoughts or feelings as clouds passing by in the sky. When you watch the clouds, you simply notice and appreciate them for what they are. You can do this with your thoughts, too! Try "sitting with them," imagining them as clouds passing by or labeling them with feeling words.

Puberty and Emotions

For example, you could say to yourself, "I know I am feeling sadness. I am going to sit with it until it goes by on its own because I know it will." Mindfulness doesn't make your thoughts or feelings go away, but it helps you accept them and enjoy the present moment instead of worrying about the past or the future.

Here's another mindfulness trick: Slowly draw your name in fun letters on a piece of paper. Pay attention to each stroke of the marker, noticing the shapes you're creating while also paying attention to your thoughts and feelings as you go along.

Find ways to practice self-care.

Self-care is what it sounds like—taking care of yourself! Here's a self-care exercise that can help you feel good about yourself:

Start by making two lists. Create one list with some of your favorite activities. It could be taking a bath, going to the movies, or eating pizza.

Make a second list with some activities that you don't always want to do but know you'd feel proud of afterward, like doing a chore or getting started on a school project.

Notice how both lists help you take care of yourself—sometimes in a fun way, other times in a way that will help your future self. Self-care sets you up to feel good tomorrow, next week, and next year.

Puberty and Emotions

Now combine each list and do one or a few self-care activities every day. Mix it up—do things from both lists. Whether practicing your favorite sport or raking the leaves in the yard, self-care activities help you feel better because you are having fun and relaxing while still taking care of your needs and responsibilities.

Use good body language.

Body language is how we hold our shoulders, the volume of our voice, the way we move our hands, and our eye contact and facial expressions. It tells others a lot about us and how we're feeling. Do you slump your shoulders when someone picks on you? Do you sit up straight and shoot up your hand when you know an answer? As you can see, body language can be positive or negative, but positive body language makes us feel better and more confident!

Here are two ways to help you become aware of body language and use it to change how you feel:

Stand in front of a mirror. Practice how you might appear if you were scared, or embarrassed, or proud. Notice how your face and posture, and body show your feelings. How can you change these to be more positive?

Practice confident body language. Try standing up straight, speaking up clearly, or doing a superhero pose in front of the mirror. And when you feel negative body language coming on, use these tricks to stand proud!

Puberty and Emotions

Seek Out a Professional

Some situations cannot be fixed by talking to a friend, practicing mindfulness, or getting a good night's sleep. There are millions of people all over the world who have mental health struggles. About half of you reading this book will need some extra support. There are a wide variety of mental health professionals to help guide you if you have concerns. Social workers, psychologists, psychiatrists, and your family doctor all have the training to help you. Your trusted adult or school counselor can help you find the right professional for you.

Here are some warning signs that you might need professional help.

Nothing brings you joy or happiness.
You feel alone and like you have no friends.
You aren't motivated to do anything.
You feel anxious or sad all the time.
You feel unsafe in your environment.
You have thoughts about harming yourself or others.

Most people don't know what to expect when they need to visit a mental health professional. In simplest terms, they are talking doctors. You should not be afraid to talk to a mental health professional or feel as if there is something wrong with you. It just means you need a little extra help.

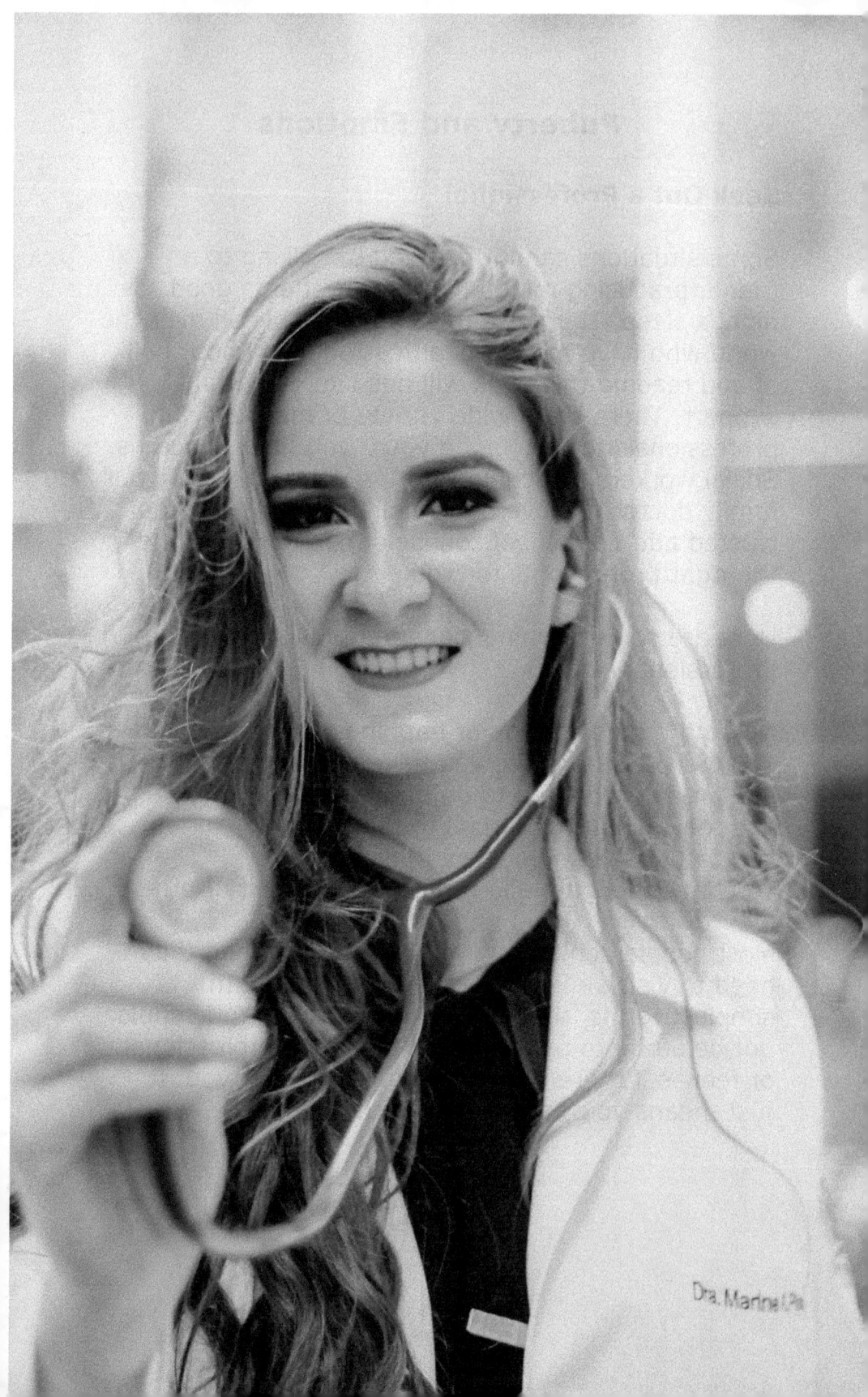

Puberty and Emotions

If you broke your arm, you would see a doctor to help you fix it. Instead of getting an arm cast in the office, you spend time in the office talking about your feelings and ways to help manage them.

Therapists are different than talking to your BFF or parents because they are not biased, are not a part of your everyday life, and are obligated to keep your information completely confidential. Your parents and friends don't have the same training as a professional. Don't hesitate to reach out for help if you need it.

Tips for Parents

Parenthood is a gift, and every mom and dad does well to be thankful for the privileges of being a parent. Being a parent to a daughter requires much love and dedication, for daughters are, indeed, special. Every time a little girl bids farewell to childhood and says hello to growing up, parents experience happiness and sadness. It is a bittersweet feeling as their little girl is finally on her way to becoming a young woman.

At this point in your child's life, you need to be a strong pillar, good model, and sound adviser. But most of all, you need to be a parent with consistent, reliable support. Be there for her. Talk to her about Puberty and sex clearly and matter-of-factly. Prepare her well for the changes up ahead. You have to make her mentally and emotionally ready. Here are valuable tips that all parents can use as they take on this responsibility.

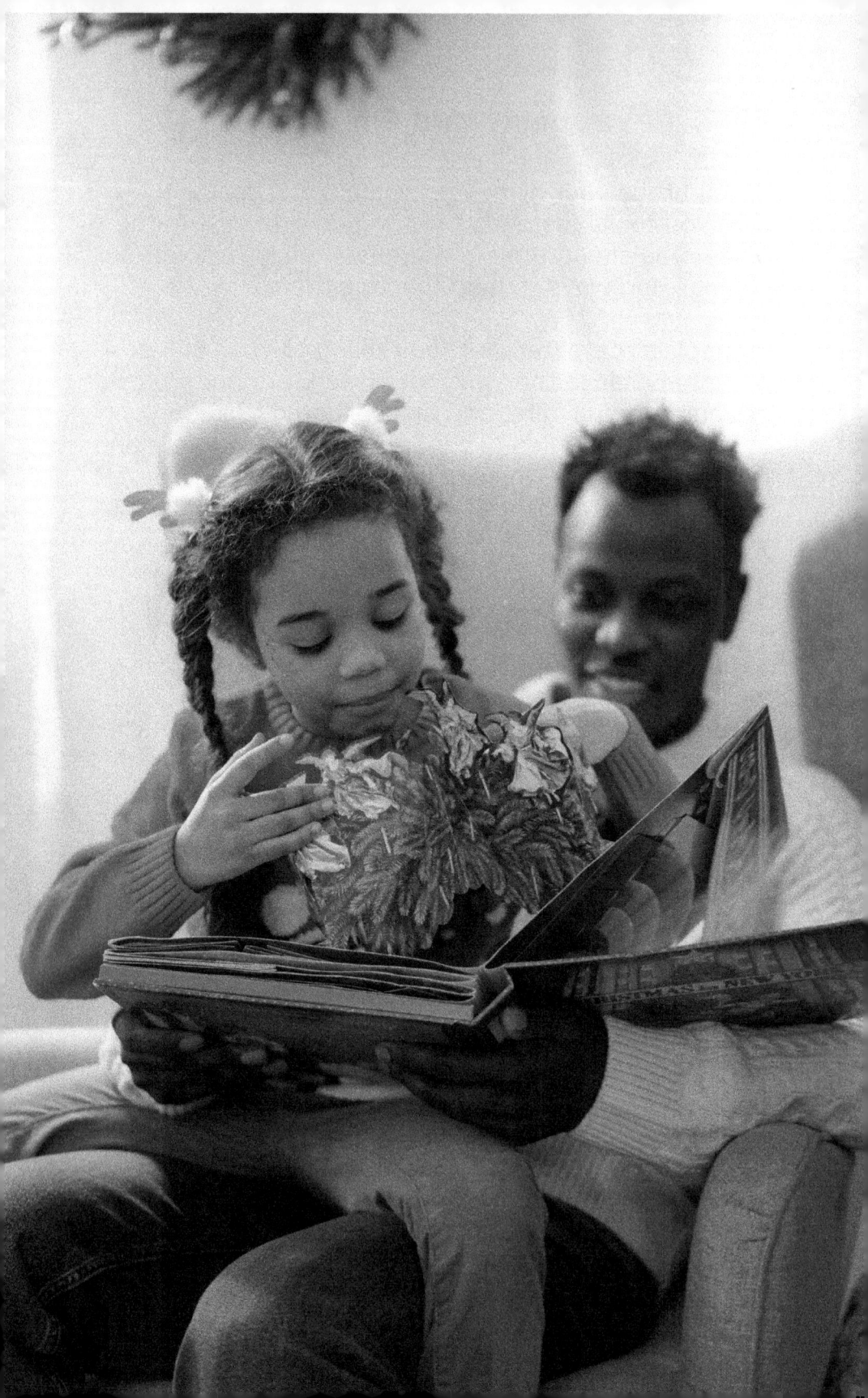

Puberty and Emotions

Tip #1: Keep Lines of Communication Open

Your child should feel that she can talk to you about anything. Create an environment where she will not feel afraid or embarrassed to ask questions. At this stage, young girls may want to talk about their feelings for boys, too, not only about the physical changes happening to their bodies.

Be sure to be ready when she opens up about a crush. Don't freak out and give a sermon about her being too young to fall in love. Instead, encourage her to speak up, be understanding, offer her support, and most importantly, give the appropriate advice.

Tip #2: Provide Honest Answers

When your daughter does ask you a question about Puberty and sex, always give an honest answer. The fact that she came to you means that she trusts you and thinks that you will be able to enlighten her. Don't evade her question, or worse, give a bogus answer.

To help you answer her questions better, first, clarify what exactly it is that she wants to know and, from this information, provide the answer that she needs. Second, answer her questions one at a time. It will help you provide the correct answers, and she will be able to absorb the new information much more effectively. Third, allow her to form her questions. Give her time to talk.

Puberty and Emotions

Don't form her questions for her, and don't jump to conclusions. By doing these three steps, you'll be able to give your daughter the answer she needs.

Tip #3: Refresh Your Knowledge

You wouldn't go to war without a weapon, would you? Having sex talk with your daughter is by no means comparable to going to war, but it would greatly help if you were prepared and knew what you were talking about. It is highly recommended that you brush up on your biology, anatomy, and physiology. You'll be able to provide more accurate and definite replies to your child's questions if you are clear with the terminology, bodily functions, and processes.

Tip #4: Make It Practical

When giving "the talk" to your child, don't let it resemble an extra biology class. You are not her teacher; you are her parent. So talk to her about menstruation, Puberty, and sex on a more personal level. Avoid sounding like you're giving her a science lecture. Give practical information that she can use in her daily life, such as keeping extra pads in her bag or school locker, what to do when her pants get stained while she's at school, and handling menstruation cramps, etc.

Puberty and Emotions

Tip #5: Stop, Talk, and Listen

Remember always to allow two-way communication. Speak and listen, listen and speak. Don't just deliver a monologue and tell her to scram. This talk is a crucial one, so make sure that you connect with your daughter. Assure her that you are always there to listen, and if she ever needs advice, she can go to you anytime.

Tip #6: Pick the Appropriate Time and Place

The best time to tell your daughter about menstruation is when she is around 8 to 9 years old. If you wait any longer, she might have her first period without knowing about it, and that could freak her out. When initiating the talk about her first period, Puberty, and sex, you must sit her down for it. Set a schedule for this talk or pick the right moment to broach the subject but remember to sit her down so that she can absorb what you will tell her.

Make sure that her siblings are not around listening and ready to make fun of her. It is also a bad idea to talk in front of her friends, family, and relatives. Your daughter considers her bedroom a safe place, and it is best to do the talk here where she will be most comfortable. Also, you can prevent interruptions and distractions.

Puberty and Emotions

There are moments between a parent and the child when they are most connected. It is the perfect time to talk to your daughter about her first period.

Finally, comfort your daughter with the knowledge that all girls and boys go through Puberty and that she isn't the only one experiencing the physical changes and overwhelming emotions. Perhaps, you can tell her that Puberty is comparable to the caterpillar stage that every butterfly has to go through. So this awkward stage in her life will pass, and she, too, will become a beautiful, confident woman when the time comes.

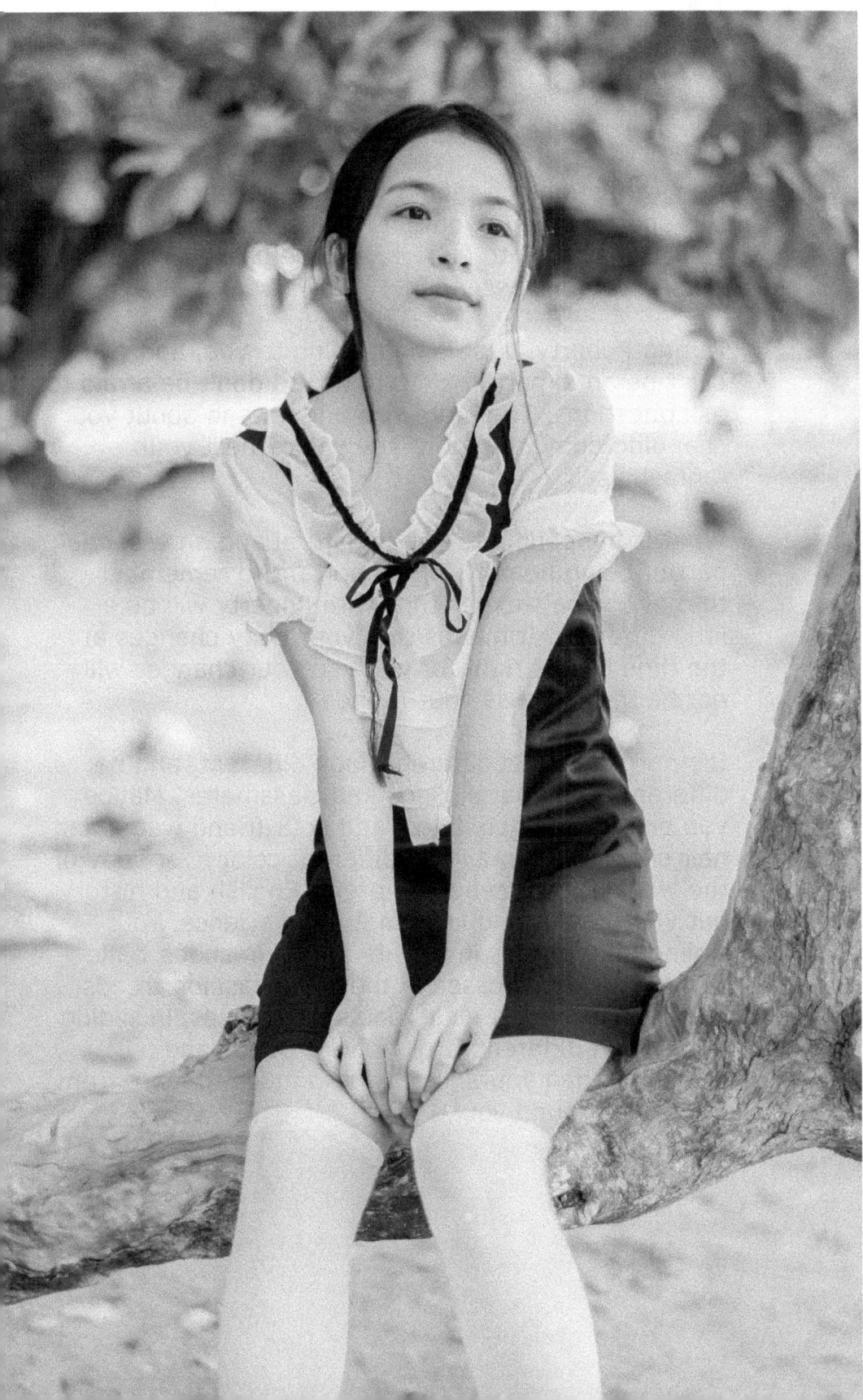

Conclusion

Congratulations on taking the time to learn about this special time in your life! You should celebrate your transition into Puberty and be proud of the person you are becoming.

During Puberty, a lot is happening to you, and you can't be an expert in everything, so don't be afraid to ask questions. The more you understand about your changing body, the more you will respect your fantastic self.

What is happening to you is natural and an essential part of being healthy. It's important to remember that everyone's experience with Puberty will be a little different. It means that your body changes at the time that is right for you—so your changes will not be the same as your friends'.

It's normal to feel different, look different, and be different than your siblings and classmates. Maybe you prefer long hairstyles, and your friend wears her hair short (and sprayed a different color every day of the week!). Or maybe you prefer English and history, but your best friend likes math and science. Your sibling might dress in sweats and gym shoes while you are always dressed in the latest fashion trends. Learn to appreciate everyone's differences, including those from different family backgrounds and traditions than yours. There is so much to learn from everyone around you!

Conclusion

You are capable and prepared to tackle adolescence and the joys and challenges it brings. Life will always have ups and downs, but by reading this book and continuing to learn about your body and brain, you will have the knowledge to tackle anything that comes your way. Surround yourself with a winning team that supports you for who you want to be.

You have learned so much about your body and all the changes you can expect over the next few years. I hope you feel more intelligent and more prepared to handle Puberty. Most of all, I hope you have learned that you are already a phenomenal girl, and Puberty can't and won't change that. If anything, Puberty can help you feel more confident and clear about what an incredible human being you are.
Be proud of yourself. Be proud of your growing body.

You have taken a big step to learn so much important information about how your body works, and the changes to come. That is the sign of a bright and capable girl committed to taking good care of herself. You are well on your way to becoming the best version of yourself. Enjoy the ride!

Finally, if you enjoyed this book, please take the time to share your thoughts and post a review on Amazon. It'd be much appreciated!

https://www.amazon.com/dp/B092467B4B
Scroll down on the left.
(Write a customer review) tab

Many Thanks!

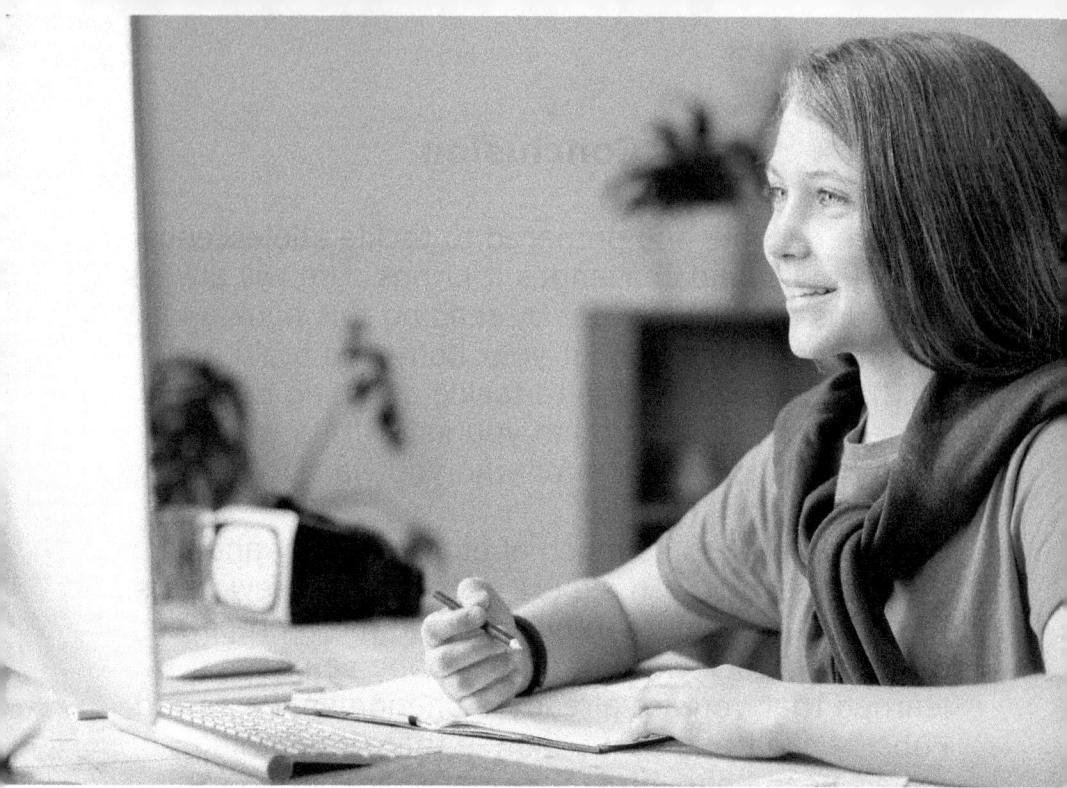

www.ingramcontent.com/pod-product-compliance
Lightning Source LLC
Chambersburg PA
CBHW060253030426
42335CB00014B/1675